Psychiatry for the Boards

Second Edition

Psychiatry for the Boards

Second Edition

William W. Wang, M.D., Ph.D.
Director of Medical Research
Advent Research Institute
Medical Director
Geriatric Transitional Program
SSM St. Joseph Health Center
St. Charles, Missouri

Wen-Hui Cai, M.D., Ph.D.
Assistant Professor of Psychiatry
University of Texas
Southwestern Medical Center at Dallas
Dallas, Texas

Wolters Kluwer | Lippincott Williams & Wilkins
Health
Philadelphia • Baltimore • New York • London
Buenos Aires • Hong Kong • Sydney • Tokyo

Publisher: Charles W. Mitchell
Developmental Editor: Jennifer LaGreca
Managing Editor: Sirkka Howes Bertling
Project Manager: Jennifer Harper
Manufacturing Coordinator: Kathleen Brown
Associate Director of Marketing: Adam Glazer
Creative Director: Doug Smock
Production Services: International Typesetting and Composition

530 Walnut Street
Philadelphia, PA 19106
LWW.com

Printed in the USA

Library of Congress Cataloging-in-Publication Data

Cai, Wen-Hui, M.D.
Psychiatry for the boards/Wen-Hui Cai, William W. Wang. —2nd ed.
p. ; cm.
Includes bibliographical references and index.
ISBN-13: 978-0-7817-7482-6
ISBN-10: 0-7817-7482-9
1. Psychiatry—Examinations, questions, etc. I. Wang, William W. II. Title.
[DNLM: 1. Psychiatry—Examination Questions. WM 18.2 C133p 2008]
RC457.C26 2008
616.890076—dc22

2007011099

Care has been taken to confirm the accuracy of the information presented and to describe generally accepted practices. However, the authors, editors, and publisher are not responsible for errors or omissions or for any consequences from application of the information in this book and make no warranty, expressed or implied, with respect to the currency, completeness, or accuracy of the contents of the publication. Application of this information in a particular situation remains the professional responsibility of the practitioner.

The authors, editors, and publisher have exerted every effort to ensure that drug selection and dosage set forth in this text are in accordance with current recommendations and practice at the time of publication. However, in view of ongoing research, changes in government regulations, and the constant flow of information relating to drug therapy and drug reactions, the reader is urged to check the package insert for each drug for any change in indications and dosage and for added warnings and precautions. This is particularly important when the recommended agent is a new or infrequently employed drug.

Some drugs and medical devices presented in this publication have Food and Drug Administration (FDA) clearance for limited use in restricted research settings. It is the responsibility of health care providers to ascertain the FDA status of each drug or device planned for use in their clinical practice.

The publisher has made every effort to trace copyright holders for borrowed material. If they have inadvertently overlooked any, they will be pleased to make the necessary arrangements at the first opportunity.

To purchase additional copies of this book, call our customer service department at (800) 638-3030 or fax orders to (301) 223-2320. International customers should call (301) 223-2300. Lippincott Williams & Wilkins customer service representatives are available from 8:30 am to 6:30 pm, EST, Monday through Friday, for telephone access. Visit Lippincott Williams & Wilkins on the Internet: http://www.lww.com.

10 9 8 7 6 5 4 3

To The Memory of Cindy—
WWW

To Fangru, David, and Mark—
WHC

Contents

Preface to the Second Edition

Psychiatry for the Boards presents a unique collection of knowledge that, to our belief, is essential for the study of clinical psychiatry. This second edition of *Psychiatry for the Boards* bears significantly enriched text and a broadened spectrum of material. This book is completely up-to-date at the time of publication. The major improvements are:

1. All the contents are updated to match DSM-IV-TR.
2. New developments in neuroscience and technology are included.
3. New psychopharmacologic agents are included.
4. Comments and suggestions from readers of the first edition, and many of them with recent experience taking the PRITE®, Board, and USMLE, are also included.
5. Over 50% of the text is revised.
6. About 40% of the chapters are completely rewritten and retitled accordingly.
7. We added six new chapters: Human Development; ECT, VNS, and DBS; Seizure Disorders; Localized Impairment: Strokes, Brain Injuries, and Brain Tumors; Peripheral Nerve and Muscle Disorders; and Cranial Nerve Symptoms and Disorders.
8. The number of sample Board-type questions has been increased from 85 to 100.

The volume has grown moderately, but we strived to keep our promise of creating a high-yield and easy-to-read book in a manageable size. We resisted the temptation of being overly inclusive and comprehensive. We understand our readers, be they physicians, residents, or medical students, are not interested in adding another mammoth volume to their bookshelves. As in our first edition, we continue to observe the principle of being concise and using plain language whenever possible. Based on our rigorous research on standard national examinations of clinical psychiatry, we are confident that the second edition continues to be a very effective test-preparation tool.

The practical tips at the end of the book also include readers' input. We are confident that the optimal use of information in this book and adherence to the study plan will significantly improve the reader's score on the PRITE, Board, and USMLE exams in a period of several weeks.

William W. Wang, M.D., Ph.D.
Wen-Hui Cai, M.D., Ph.D.

PART I

BASIC KNOWLEDGE

CHAPTER 1 Psychosocial Theories and Behavioral Sciences

What is attachment?

Attachment is the emotional and behavioral dependence of an infant to its primary caregiver. It involves the senses of resources and security.

Attachment develops between the ages of 6 to 8 weeks and 3 years, and lasts for life.

Attachment theory was developed by John Bowlby.

What is "bonding"?

The term "bonding" is often used alternatively for attachment. However, bonding is not associated with resources and security (e.g., a mother feels anxious but does not feel unsafe when she is separated from her infant).

Attachment: Child → Mother

Bonding: Mother → Child

Insecure attachments may be associated with the development of personality disorders.

What is the "strange situation"?

Developed by Mary Ainsworth in the mid-1980s, "strange situation" is a research protocol for assessing an infant's attachment.

What is classical conditioning?

Also called "respondent conditioning," classical conditioning results from the repeated pairing of a neutral (conditioned) stimulus with one that evokes a response (unconditioned stimulus), such that the neutral stimulus eventually comes to evoke the response.

Give an example of Pavlov classical conditioning.

Example: A dog salivated when it had food in its mouth, saw the food, smelled the food, or even when it heard the footsteps of a person coming to feed it.

Food: Unconditioned stimulus (UCS).

Food → salivation: Unconditioned response (UCR).

Footsteps: Conditioned stimulus (CS).

Footsteps → salivation: Conditioned response (CR).

The concept of classical conditioning was developed by Ivan Pavlov.

In classical conditioning theory, what are extinction, generalization, and discrimination?

Extinction: When a CS is repeated without being paired with its UCS, the CR gradually weakens and eventually disappears. However, the UCR does not become extinct.

Generalization: The transferring of a CS from one stimulus to another. A dog may respond to the footsteps of people other than its feeder, or even to noises other than footsteps. Transference during psychotherapy was explained as stimulus generalization.

Discrimination: Recognizing and responding to differences between similar stimuli. A smart dog knows when its feeder is coming.

How does one maintain a behavior so that it is resistant to extinction?

Give the positive reinforcement intermittently, and in a variable-ratio schedule.

Mechanism of extinction applied to substance-related disorders:

CS (conditioned stimulus): Environment associated with craving.

UCS (unconditioned stimulus): Drug.

CR (conditioned response): Craving.

The CR was established with repeated exposure to a paired UCS and CS. When the patient is repeatedly exposed to an unpaired CS (i.e., when a UCS is not available), the craving may finally become extinct.

What is operant conditioning?

It is a form of learning in which behavioral frequency is altered through the application of positive and negative consequences. Operant conditioning is also known as "instrumental conditioning."

Example: A dog receives food only when it responds correctly by pressing a lever.

Food: Reinforcing stimulus.

Lever: Operant.

The concept of operant conditioning was developed by B.F. Skinner.

Reinforcement.

Positive reinforcement: Increases the probability that a response will recur.

Negative reinforcement: Leads to the removal of a response.

Variable-interval schedule: Reinforcement occurs at variable intervals.

State-dependent learning.

Recall of information is facilitated by the same environment in which the information was first acquired.

One may do better in an examination by wearing the same earplugs as those worn when studying for the examination.

According to Eric Erikson, what is the developmental task between the ages of 40 and 60?

This stage is the seventh stage in Erikson's life-cycle theory. Adults at this stage must choose between generativity and stagnation (cessation of growth, becoming stale). A successful choice in the developmental task is generativity (i.e., becoming useful to society through behaviors that protect future generations).

Eric Erikson's eight stages of the life cycle are:

1. *Basic trust versus basic mistrust (0 to 1 years).*
2. *Autonomy versus shame and doubt (1 to 3 years).*
3. *Initiative versus guilt (3 to 5 years).*
4. *Industry versus inferiority (6 to 11 years).*
5. *Identity versus role confusion (11 to 20 years).*
6. *Intimacy versus self-absorption or isolation (21 to 40 years).*

7. *Generativity versus stagnation (40 to 65 years).*
8. *Integrity versus despair and isolation (65 years and older).*

What are characteristic features of Eric Erikson's stage of industry versus inferiority? To which of Sigmund Freud's stages of psychosexual development does this stage correspond?

In Erikson's stage of industry versus inferiority (6 to 11 years), children are busy building, creating, and accomplishing. They are able to set up clubs with complicated rules and rituals. They also face the danger of a sense of inadequacy and inferiority. This stage corresponds to Freud's latency stage (5 to 12 years).

What is sublimation?

Sublimation is a defense mechanism through which unhealthy or unacceptable drives and affects are transformed into healthy and creative behavior.

What is conventional morality?

Conventional morality is one of the major levels of morality development. Integrating Jean Piaget's cognitive development theory, Lawrence Kohlberg described three major levels of morality:

1. Preconventional: To obey and to avoid punishment.
2. Conventional: To gain approval from others, especially peers.
3. Principle: To comply with ethical principles.

What are the principal concepts in Carol Gilligan's model of morality?

Carol Gilligan believes that there are alternate pathways to the same moral pinnacle. She proposed that girls have a greater sense of connection and concern with relationships than with rules (i.e., that girls rely on intuitive sense in decision making).

According to modern psychodynamic theory, what factors are the most important in the formation of adult personality?

The most important factors are:

1. Inherited traits.
2. Environment.
3. Experiences of infancy and childhood.

What is "learned helplessness"?

It is an animal model of depression. After a period of intermittent electric shocks from which there is no possible escape, the animal gave up further attempts to escape from the shocks.

The concept of learned helplessness was developed by Martin Seligman and is a well-recognized model of an experimental depressive disorder. The apparent cessation of efforts to escape from shock becomes generalized to other situations, and eventually the animal always becomes helpless and apathetic.

Primary process versus secondary process.

According to Sigmund Freud, primary-process thinking is the primitive form of cognitive activity that is motivated by the pleasure principle.

Primary-process thinking is revised by the ego to become coherent, mature, and rational. This revision is called the secondary process or secondary revision, and is guided by the reality principle.

What is anal fixation?

According to classic psychoanalytic theory, anal fixation is a form of regression in response to castration anxiety encountered in the oedipal phase. Anally-fixated persons are viewed as victims of a harsh and strict superego.

What personality disorder has its development associated with anal fixation?

The characteristic pattern of anal fixation includes excessive orderliness, perseverance, emotional constriction, a tendency to intellectualize, indecisiveness, procrastination, and stubbornness. All of these features are characteristic for obsessive-compulsive personality disorder.

What are the psychosexual developmental stages in Sigmund Freud's theory?

The stages of psychosexual development set forth in Sigmund Freud's theory are:

1. *Oral (birth to 18 months).*
2. *Anal (1 to 3 years).*
3. *Phallic (oedipal, 3 to 5 years).*
4. *Latency (5 to 12 years).*
5. *Genital (12 years to adulthood).*

What is psychic determinism?

One of the principal beliefs of psychoanalysis is that behavior has meaning. A particular behavior is determined by "psychic" motivation in the form of unconscious drives, defenses, object relationships, and self-disturbances. A central feature of psychic determinism is that childhood experiences are repeated throughout life.

What are the basics of Salvador Minuchin's theory of family system and family therapy?

Salvador Minuchin was one of the early conceptualists of the family system, and the originator of structural family therapy.

Structural family therapy focuses on the current organization (structure) of a family.

Analysis of interactions (between family members, in therapeutic sessions) allows the therapist to clarify how the family's organization influences (promotes or inhibits) task performance, especially child-rearing.

The therapist promotes those interactions that introduce greater flexibility, alternative patterns and structures, and more effective task performance.

Minuchin's form of family therapy was developed to address child and adolescent emotional and behavioral problems, and is particularly effective in such situations. It is arguably the most influential form of family therapy.

On the basis of Salvador Minuchin's theory of family interactions, explain the phenomenon of a mother constantly staying with her ill son and calling his disease "our disease."

Enmeshment (ineffective closeness) and disengagement (excessive distance), as well as rapid fluctuations between interactional extremes, are manifestations of dysfunctional family relationships.

Other core concepts of Minuchin's theory include boundaries, hierarchies, coalitions, alliances, and complementarity.

The case described above, of the mother remaining with her ill son, is a typical case of enmeshment.

What did Stephen Suomi's studies of the total isolation of infant monkeys imply?

These studies implied that "therapist" monkeys could help socialize infants.

In 1972, Stephen Suomi demonstrated that monkey isolates could be rehabilitated if they were exposed to monkeys that promote physical contact without threatening the isolates with aggression or overly complex play interactions. These monkeys were called therapist monkeys. To fill such a therapeutic role, Suomi chose young normal monkeys that played gently with the isolates and would approach and cling to them. Within 2 weeks, the isolates were reciprocating the social contact, and their incidence of abnormal self-directed behaviors began to decline significantly. By the end of a 6-month treatment period, the isolates were actively initiating play bouts with both the therapist monkeys and each other, and most of their self-directed behaviors had disappeared. Two years later, the isolates' improved behavior had not regressed.

CHAPTER 2 Human Development

According to whose theory is good-enough mothering important in providing a supportive environment to infants?

Good-enough mothering is an essential concept in Donald W. Winnicott's object-relation theory.

Another important concept of Winnicott's theory is that of the transitional object.

At what age do children with Tourette syndrome start to present with symptoms?

Between 6 and 10 years.

At what age does stranger anxiety develop?

Stranger anxiety is first noted at the age of 7 months, and develops fully at the age of 8 months.

What are the basics of Heinz Kohut's theory of personality?

Individuals (selves) need empathic interaction with their mother and the other family members (objects).

This interaction is called self-object function.

Failure of self-object function may lead to developmental arrest and personality disorders.

What are the characteristics of Jean Piaget's concrete operational stage?

Rational and logical thought.

The concept of conservation (water in a tall cup has the same volume as water in a bowl).

The ability to understand someone else's point of view.

What are the characteristics of Piaget's sensorimotor stage?

Occurs from birth to 2 years of age.

Stereotyped reaction to stimuli.

Object permanency.

What are the characteristics of the preoperational stage?

Symbolic functions.

Egocentric thinking.

Magical thinking.

Basic moral thought.

At what age does a child begin to preferentially look and listen to the mother?

One week.

What are the cognitive developmental characteristics in the formal operational stage of Jean Piaget's theory of development?

Beyond 11 years of age, an individual is able to deal with concepts and ideas.

This pattern of thinking and reasoning is described as abstract, deductive, and conceptual.

Synthesis, the integration of traits, attitudes, and impulses to create a total personality, is an important task in this stage.

What are the first signs of onset of puberty in girls?

Pubic hair growth.

Breast enlargement.

What is a transitional object?

An infant's "not-me" possession, usually a reassuring blanket or toy, that preserves the illusion of the comforting maternal object even in her absence.

The term "transitional object" was coined by Donald W. Winnicott.

At what age do children start to understand that death is permanent?

Seven years.

What is infantile amnesia?

Most people cannot recall events that happened before 5 years of age.

This phenomenon is probably caused by the lack of language-based retrieval of prelinguistic memory.

What is introjection?

Internalizing the qualities of an object, as in the case of a child mentally incorporating a model of his mother as a soothing presence.

What is priming?

Priming is facilitation of the ability to identify stimuli on the basis of recent experience with the same stimuli.

Example: Amnestic patients may show a normal tendency to complete three-letter stems on the basis of previously encountered words.

What is the difference between declarative memory and nondeclarative memory?

Declarative memory:

- Also known as explicit memory.
- Requires conscious awareness and concentration.

- Impaired after brain injury.
- Deals with facts and events.
- Brain structures include hippocampus, orbitofrontal cortex (overlapping with nondeclarative memory), and parahippocampal gyrus.

Nondeclarative memory:

- Also known as implicit memory.
- Cannot be expressed in words.
- Does not require focal, conscious attention.
- Usually remains intact after brain injury.
- Deals with skills (procedural), habits, priming, simple classical conditioning, and nonassociative learning.
- Brain structures include basal ganglia, limbic system (amygdala, anterior cingulate gyrus, and orbitofrontal cortex), and perceptual cortices.

What is the first physical change during female sexual development?

A growth spurt in height.

What is the psychoanalytic explanation for adolescents' unreasoning passion about celebrity stars and cult figures?

In psychoanalytic theory, it is believed that this phenomenon is related to the direction of adolescents' feelings away from parents, and their unconscious displacement of incestuous thoughts.

What is the stage at which a child with a congenital physical deformity is most vulnerable to emotional disturbance?

Early adolescence or age 11 to 15 years.

What is egocentrism?

Children see themselves as the center of the universe. They are unable to take the role of another person.

Example: A child holds a picture facing toward himself and asks the mother about items in the picture, not realizing that the mother can only see the back of the picture.

A characteristic feature of children in the preoperational stage (2 to 7 years).

A term used in Jean Piaget's developmental theory. Jean Piaget's developmental stages are:

Sensorimotor (0 to 2 years).

Preoperational (2 to 7 years).

Concrete operational (7 to 11 years).

Formal operational (11 years onward).

What type of memory deals with skill and habits?

Implicit memory (nondeclarative memory).

When does gender identity become fixed?

At the age of 2 to 3 years.

When does the synaptogenesis of neuronal circuitry during brain development reach its peak?

At the toddler stage (2 to 3 years).

What is rapprochement?

The fifth developmental stage in Margaret Mahler's separation-individuation theory.

This French word means "reconciliation."

In the stage of rapprochement, children are constantly concerned about the actual physical location of their mothers, and have great need for maternal love.

Lack of maternal love or absence of the mother during the rapprochement stage may lead to a child's temper tantrums, whining, and moodiness, and has been linked to the pathogenesis of borderline personality disorder.

CHAPTER 3

Psychometric and Neuropsychologic Testing

What is the best psychologic test to use for assessing possible malingering?

Arguably, the Minnesota Multiphasic Personality Inventory (MMPI), since it has a built-in test detecting inconsistent responses.

A patient scores very low in WAIS-R subtests for picture arrangement and block design as compared to other subtests. What does this result suggest?

WAIS-R: Wechsler Adult Intelligence Scale—Revised, developed by David Wechsler, a Romanian American psychologist;

A disproportionately low score in picture arrangement and block design implies a lesion in the nondominant hemisphere.

What are SCID and MINI?

SCID: The Structured Clinical Interview for the DSM-IV;

A semistructured interview that applies DSM-IV criteria;

Administered by a clinician, is time-consuming, and is therefore used only in research;

Arguably the most reliable instrument for diagnosing psychiatric disorders.

MINI: The Mini-International Neuropsychiatric Interview;

Similar to SCID but more compact and demands only yes/no answers rather than those shown on a numerical scale.

What does the Millon Clinical Multiaxial Inventory-II assess?

It measures personality styles, expressed concerns, and behavioral correlates.

What is the Bender Gestalt Test?

Also known as the Bender Gestalt Visual-Motor Test.

Assesses visuomotor integration and visual construction.

Originally designed to measure maturational levels in children, the test may also suggest some deficiency in construction ability.

Signs of brain damage on the Bender Gestalt Test include visual neglect, rotation of designs, perseveration, and distorted designs.

What is MMPI-2?

Minnesota Multiphasic Personality Inventory-2, a revision of the original MMPI.

A self-report inventory, one of the most widely used and thoroughly researched objective instruments for personality assessment.

It contains more than 500 statements and gives scores on 10 standard clinical scales.

It is used to identify major areas of psychopathologic functioning.

What is the Brief Psychotic Rating Scale (BPRS)?

A psychometric instrument;

Used to assess quantitative severity of symptoms for schizophrenia and other psychotic disorders.

What is the major difference between Hamilton Rating Scale for Depression and Beck Depression Inventory?

HAM-D: Hamilton Rating Scale for Depression;

BDI: Beck Depression Inventory;

Both quantify the degree of depression, and are therefore useful for measuring the progress of treatment;

Neither provides diagnosis;

HAM-D is administered by the clinician;

BDI is a self-rating scale;

BDI correlates well with the HAM-D score.

What is the difference between reliability and validity?

Reliability: Refers to reproducibility. A reliable scale should provide consistent information when tested at different times and by different raters.

Validity: Refers to a scale's ability to measure what it intends to measure.

What is the Halstead-Reitan Neuropsychologic Battery and what does it measure?

Using a noninvasive psychologic test, it examines the location and effects of specific brain lesions.

It contains 10 tests:

1. Category;
2. Tactile performance;

3. Perception of rhythm;
4. Finger-oscillation;
5. Perception of speech-sounds;
6. Trail-making;
7. Perception of critical flicker frequency;
8. Time sense;
9. Aphasia screening;
10. Sensory-perceptual function.

It can be used to differentiate among early dementia, mild delirium, and depression.

What is the most widely used scale for obsessive-compulsive disorder (OCD)?

Y-BOCS: Yale-Brown Obsessive-Compulsive Scale;

Assessing the severity of OCD.

What is the Thematic Apperception Test (TAT)?

Developed by Murray and Morgan;

Used to test nonpathologic personality traits;

The testee is asked to tell a story after viewing a series of ambiguous pictures.

What is the purpose of projective testing?

To detect the presence of subtle psychotic thought processes and bizarre ideation.

Commonly used projective tests:

Rorschach Test;

Thematic Apperception Test;

Sentence Completion Test;

Word-Association Test;

Draw-A-Person Test.

What tests should be recommended to assess executive function?

Trail-making tests (e.g., the patient is requested to give sequentially alternating numbers and letters: 1-Z-2-Y-3-X . . .). These tests require rapid and efficient visual-motor integration, attention, and cognitive sequencing.

Card-sorting tests (e.g., Wisconsin Card Sorting Test [WCST]).

CHAPTER 4 Epidemiology, Biostatistics, and Social Psychiatry

What is a cohort study?

A cohort study is a study that follows a group of subjects chosen from a well-defined population over an extended period. It is a form of prospective study.

Cohort study (also known as a follow-up study): A group of individuals (cohort) is defined on the basis of having or lacking exposure to a suspected risk factor for a disease, and is followed for an extended period.

What are Case-control study, Descriptive study, and Intervention study?

Case-control study: Subjects are selected on the basis of whether they do or do not have the particular disease being studied.

Descriptive studies (including correlation studies, case reports or case series, and cross-sectional surveys): Describe patterns of disease occurrence in relation to selected variables (e.g., person, place, and time).

Intervention study: The investigator controls the allocation of subjects to different comparison groups and regulates the experimental conditions for each group.

What research design is necessary to establish a causal inference for an observed effect?

A control group study.

Construct validity.

Construct validity is the ability of a test to measure what it is designed to assess.

Reliability is the repeatability of the findings of an assessment instrument.

What is the most important factor in deciding the validity of a worker's compensation case?

A causal link between an occurrence at work and subsequent illness.

What do the sensitivity and specificity of a test measure?

Sensitivity measures the ability of a test to identify true-positive cases. Specificity measures the ability of a test to identify true-negative cases.

What is sensitivity?

The proportion of positive test results among the test group of individuals who actually have a particular condition.

Racial differences in pharmacokinetics.

Racial differences in pharmacokinetics are usually based on differences in liver enzymes.

For example, lithium is not metabolized in the liver, there are therefore few racial differences in its metabolism.

Regression analysis.

A procedure for predicting the value or behavior of one variable (the dependent variable) on the basis of the value or behavior of another variable (the independent variable). For example, one may predict a student's performance in college (X) on the basis of the student's score on a scholastic aptitude test (Y).

Y is a known value, and is the independent variable.

X is an unknown value but is somehow dependent upon Y, and is therefore the dependent variable.

In recent years, the suicide rate has increased in which population group?

Since 1960, suicide has increased dramatically among adolescents.

What is the best factor for predicting suicide?

The best factor for predicting suicide is the subject's past suicidal behavior.

What is the "drift hypothesis?"

The drift hypothesis states that disabling conditions tend to cause downward social mobility. This hypothesis offered one of the explanations for the early finding that schizophrenia and other mental disorders were more prevalent among people of low socioeconomic status.

What factors have caused an increased need for geriatric long-term mental health care?

The increase in size of the geriatric population and the lack of family supports are two important factors in the increased need for geriatric long-term mental health care.

What factors are associated with the seeking of psychiatric help?

Gender, social class, and education.

Gender: More women than men seek psychiatric help.

Social class: People of higher social class are more likely to use psychiatric services.

Education: Higher education is associated with more frequent use of psychiatric services.

What is the most common method for completed suicide among adolescents?

Use of a gun.

What type of prevention is demonstrated by abstinence from alcohol during pregnancy?

Primary prevention.

Primary prevention: Preventing the onset of a disease and thereby reducing its incidence by eliminating the causative agents, reducing risk factors, enhancing host resistance, and interfering with transmission of the disease.

Secondary prevention: Early identification and prompt treatment of an illness, with the goal of reducing its prevalence by reducing its duration.

Tertiary prevention: Reducing the prevalence of residual defects and disabilities caused by an illness; this enables those with chronic mental illnesses to reach the highest feasible level of function.

Give an example of tertiary prevention.

Enabling persons with severe, persistent mental illness to reach their highest level of functioning.

What type of prevention is involved in helping schizophrenia patients to attain their maximal level of functioning?

Tertiary prevention.

Prevalence versus incidence.

Prevalence is the proportion of individuals with existing disease at a point in time (point prevalence) or during a period of time (period prevalence).

Incidence is the proportion of individuals developing new disease during a defined period of time.

Prevalence refers to all persons who are diseased.

Incidence refers only to new cases.

There is no such thing as "point incidence."

How should one select a statistical test for evaluating the significance of a finding?

Step one: Know the type of data to be tested. The appropriate choice of a statistical test depends upon the type of data to which it is to be applied.

Step two: Choose the right test for the type of data to be tested.

What are the different types of data?

There are four types of data: Nominal, ordinal, interval, and ratio.

Nominal data are groups with no ordering (e.g., 25 males, 171 treatment respondents, 6 counties). Nominal data cannot be used to generate means and standard deviations.

Ordinal data are groups in rank order (e.g., class standing, personal preferences).

Interval data are data measured on a scale of equal intervals (e.g., temperature, height, dosage, weight). Interval data can be used to generate means and standard deviations.

A ratio is a comparison between interval data and a true or zero point (e.g., suicide rate, disease prevalence).

Nominal and interval data are frequently tested in psychiatry residency in-training examination (PRITE®) and the Board. For statistical purposes, ratio data are treated like interval data. Ordinal data are rarely used.

What are the commonly used statistical tests in psychiatric research?

Five types of statistical tests are commonly used in psychiatric research: The T-test, Chi-square test, analysis of variance (ANOVA), Pearson's coefficient correlation, and regression.

If only interval data are being used, Pearson's coefficient correlation (to reveal a linear association) or regression analysis (to reveal a nonlinear nature of the relationship) should be applied.

If only nominal data are being used, the Chi-square test should be applied.

If combined interval and nominal data are being used, and two groups of data are being compared, the T-test should be used. If more than two groups of data are being compared, ANOVA should be used.

What is meta-analysis?

Meta-analysis is a procedure that combines results from a number of similarly designed studies to estimate the effect of a variable by incorporating the information provided by all the studies.

What psychiatric illness is most frequently related to completed suicide?

Major depression.

What is standard deviation?

The degree of spread of values around the mean.

What does a *p* value of 0.05 mean?

The probability of obtaining the result by chance alone is 1:20 (5%).

Based on epidemiologic studies (National Institute of Mental Health Epidemiological Catchment Area Study), what mental illness is more likely in a male population?	Substance abuse.
What mental illnesses are more likely in a female population?	*Major depression, borderline personality, panic disorder.*
What mental illnesses are not favored in populations of either gender?	*Schizophrenia and bipolar I affective disorder.*
What is the most common cause of death among African American male youths?	Homicide.
What is the most frequently reported child abuse in the United States?	Child neglect.
National Alliance for the Mentally Ill.	Members: Families and relatives of patients. Goal: To improve patient services and research.
Psychiatric service models.	Assertive community treatment: Active outreach to patients. Traditional social work: Helps patients connect to existing services.

What is reparative therapy? What is the standpoint of the American Psychiatric Association (APA) on this issue?

A variety of psychotherapeutic approaches were developed from the 1950s to 1970s to "repair" the sexual orientation of homosexual persons.

Since the 1970s, the APA has held the position that homosexuality is a nonpathologic human potential rather than a disorder. No existing evidence supports or advises reparative therapy for it.

What is the most common mistaken diagnosis that psychiatrists make in African American patients who have major depression or bipolar disorder?

Schizophrenia.

What is the most characteristic manifestation of depression in Chinese American patients, and how should it be approached?

Chinese American patients with depression tend to have many somatic complaints, and should be approached with direct questions about mood symptoms.

What do Japanese American female patients commonly do to make their stories discrepant from collateral information when presenting with a depressive history?

They seek to minimize their distress in front of an authority figure.

What does it mean when a third-party payer says that it offers parity in mental health treatment?

Parity in this case means that mental health services are covered on a par with other health services.

What did the National Institute of Mental Health Epidemiological Catchment Area study indicate about depression in younger and older cohorts?

It showed that depression now occurs at an earlier age than it previously did, and at an increased rate as compared with the past.

CHAPTER 5 Neuroscience

How and where is serotonin synthesized?

Synthesized from precursor tryptophan.

Synthesized in axon terminal (bouton).

Cell bodies mainly in median and dorsal raphe nuclei.

The rate-limiting factor is availability of tryptophan.

How is glutamate synthesized and deactivated?

Precursors are presynaptic glucose and glutamine.

Synaptic action is terminated through reuptake.

Glutamate release is stimulated by nicotine.

How are synaptic dopamine and norepinephrine deactivated?

Dopamine and norepinephrine are deactivated in the same pathways: Either through reuptake or synaptic metabolism by monoamine oxidase-A (MAO-A) or catecholamine O-methyl transferase (COMT).

Dopamine is metabolized into homovanillic acid (HVA) by MAO-A in the synaptic cleft, or by COMT in the presynaptic neuron after reuptake.

COMT inhibitors such as entacapone are used to increase bioavailability of levodopa in the treatment of Parkinson disease.

How is the synaptic action of serotonin terminated?

Reuptake or MAO-A metabolism.

Metabolite is 5-hydroxyindoleacetic acid (5-HIAA).

In what brain location is norepinephrine synthesized?

Locus ceruleus in the upper pons.

What are excitatory receptors?

Receptors that when activated, can cause depolarization and increase the likelihood of an action potential.

Examples include: Dopamine (D1, D5), cholinergic receptors, norepinephrine (NE-α1, NE-β), serotonin (5-HT1c, 5-HT2, 5-HT3), glutamate receptors, and substance P-NK.

What are G-protein coupled receptors?

A membrane anchored receptor with a single unit.

A single peptide forms seven transmembrane domains.

They use a second messenger system, therefore are slow in response.

Examples of G-protein coupled receptors: All 5-HT receptors except 5-HT3, most dopamine receptors, all opioid receptors, norepinephrine receptors.

What are inhibitory receptors?

Receptors that when activated, can cause hyperpolarization and decrease the likelihood of an action potential.

Examples include: Dopamine D2, D3, D4, NE-α2, 5-HT1A, γ-aminobutyric acid (GABA-A), opioid μ and δ.

What are ligand gated ion channels?

Ion channels connected to a receptor. The binding of ligands to the receptor changes the opening of the ion channels, and therefore regulates the ion channels.

What are major locations of dopamine-producing neurons in the central nervous system?

Substantia nigra, supplies nigrostriatal pathway, associated with extrapyramidal syndrome;

Ventral tegmental area (VTA), supplies mesolimbic pathway and mesocortical pathway, associated with antipsychotic effects and reward system;

Hypothalamus, supplies tuberoinfundibular pathway, associated with prolactin regulation.

It is generally assumed that the mesolimbic pathway is associated with positive symptoms, and the mesocortical pathway is associated with negative symptoms.

What are major peptide neurotransmitters in the central nervous system (CNS)?

Endogenous opioids (enkephalins, endorphins, and dynorphins).

Substance P.
Neurotensin.
Somatostatin.
Vasopressin.
Oxytocin.
Neuropeptide Y.

All peptide neurotransmitters are synthesized in the soma (cell body).

All receptors for peptide neurotransmitters are G-protein coupled, and have seven transmembrane domains.

What are the characteristics of dopamine receptors?

Dopamine receptors are all G-protein coupled receptors.

There are five subtypes.

D1 and D5 are excitatory receptors. When activated, D1 and D5 increase cyclic adenosine monophosphate (cAMP) formation.

D2, D3, and D4 are inhibitory receptors. When activated, they inhibit cAMP formation.

What are the characteristics of histamine receptors?

There are three types of histamine receptors: H1, H2, and H3.

Stimulation of H1 may increase the production of inositol 1,4,5-trisphosphate (IP3) and diacylglycerol (DAG). Blockade of H1 receptors produces relief of allergic reactions, and may cause hypotension, sedation, and weight gain.

Blockade of H2 receptors can decrease gastric acid production.

H3 is involved in regulation of the vascular system.

What are the characteristics of the rate-limiting enzyme for GABA synthesis?

Glutamic acid decarboxylase.

This enzyme utilizes pyridoxine (vitamin B6) as a cofactor.

GABA is synthesized only in the CNS, and it does not cross the blood–brain barrier.

What are the major inhibitory and excitatory neurotransmitters?

Excitatory neurotransmitter: Glutamate;

Inhibitory neurotransmitters: GABA and glycine.

What are the mechanisms of glutamate action on N-methyl-D-aspartate (NMDA) sites?

NMDA receptor is a ligand gated Ca^{2+} ion channel.

Activation of NMDA receptors causes influx of Ca^{2+}.

Activation of NMDA receptors requires two molecules of glutamate and one of glycine bound to the receptor.

Mg^{2+} and phencyclidine block the ion channel.

Proper regulation of NMDA receptors plays a key role in learning and memory.

Dysregulation of NMDA receptors is associated with psychosis and dementia. Excessive stimulation of NMDA receptors causes excitotoxicity and results in neuronal apoptosis.

What are the rate-limiting enzymes for glycine synthesis?

The synthesis of the inhibitory neurotransmitter glycine is required to create rate-limiting enzymes.

Serine transhydroxy-methylase.

B-glycerate dehydrogenase.

What illicit drugs act on the CNS dopamine receptor system?

Amphetamine stimulates dopamine release.

Cocaine inhibits dopamine reuptake.

What illicit drugs exert their effects through the serotonergic system?

Lysergic acid diethylamide is a serotonergic and dopaminergic stimulant.

Ecstasy (methylenedioxymethamphetamine or MDMA) is a potent blocker of serotonin reuptake.

What is excitotoxicity?

Excessive stimulation of glutamate receptors leads to excessive calcium influx into cells.

This may lead to protease activation, and cause apoptosis (programmed cell death).

This is proposed to be the mechanism of neuronal damage in psychosis and other psychiatric as well as neurologic diseases.

How does melatonin regulate day and night cycles (circadian cycles)?

Melatonin is a neurohormone secreted by the pineal gland.

Binds to melatonin receptors at the suprachiasmatic nucleus in the hypothalamus, and regulates circadian function.

Melatonin's action is inhibited by the input from the retinohypothalamic tract. At the end of the day, when the inhibitory input from the retinohypothalamic tract decreases, the secretion of melatonin increases.

What is substance P?

A neurotransmitter associated with pain perception.

It primarily appears in afferent sensory neurons and the nigrostriatal pathway.

What is the central nervous reward system?

It is a peptide neurotransmitter.

A neuropsychologic system associated with feelings of reward and satisfaction.

It is hypothesized to be associated with the mesolimbic and mesocortical dopamine pathways.

This is thought to be the primary neurophysiologic mechanism of addiction.

What is the chemical nature of endogenous opioids?

Peptide neurotransmitters.

Bind to opioid receptors. There are three major types of opioid receptors: δ, κ, and μ.

Enkephalins bind δ receptors.

Endorphins bind δ and μ receptors.

Dynorphins bind μ and κ receptors.

What is the endocrinologic effect of dopamine?

Dopamine inhibits the release of prolactin through the tuberoinfundibular pathway.

What are the characteristics and function of GABA receptors?

Membrane-anchored receptors.

Chloride channels.

Regulated by GABA and many other ligands.

When activated, they open the Cl^- channels and allow more Cl^- influx, and therefore increase the membrane polarization (i.e., there is higher negative charge inside the cell).

Benzodiazepines and many nonbenzodiazepine agents bind to specific sites on GABA receptors and facilitate the effects of GABA (i.e., increase the affinity of the GABA receptors to GABA).

Nonbenzodiazepine agents include zolpidem (Ambien), zaleplon (Sonata), and eszopiclone (Lunesta).

What is the rate-limiting step in dopamine synthesis?

From tyrosine to DOPA, catalyzed by tyrosine hydroxylase.

This reaction occurs in the presynaptic bouton of the dopamine neuron.

What is the rate-limiting enzyme in dopamine synthesis?

Tyrosine hydroxylase.

What is the rate-limiting step in norepinephrine synthesis?

From tyrosine to DOPA, the same step as in dopamine synthesis.

The rate-limiting enzyme is tyrosine hydroxylase.

Dopamine hydroxylase converts dopamine to norepinephrine.

What is the significance of a low 5-HIAA level in cerebrospinal fluid?

It is associated with:

Aggressive behavior;

Suicide by violent methods.

Where are neurotransmitters synthesized?

Most neurotransmitters are synthesized in the presynaptic axon terminal, also known as the bouton.

Peptide neurotransmitters are synthesized in the cell body, also known as the soma.

Where are serotonin-producing neurons located?

Raphe nuclei, located in the upper pons and midbrain;

Caudal locus ceruleus (to a lesser extent).

Where is the brain location for histamine synthesis?

Hypothalamus.

Where is the CNS location of acetylcholine-producing neurons?

Nucleus basalis of Meynert located at the basal forebrain.

Neuronal loss in this area was found in those with Alzheimer disease.

Which neurotransmitters influence aggressive behavior?

Induction of aggression: Dopamine;

Inhibition of aggression: Norepinephrine, serotonin, GABA;

The levels of 5-HIAA (serotonin's major metabolite) in cerebrospinal fluid inversely correlates with the frequency of aggression.

PART II

CLINICAL PSYCHIATRY

CHAPTER 6 Psychiatric Interview, Symptomatology, and Diagnosis

What is delusion?

It is fixed, false belief that is unreal, idiosyncratic, and not accepted by other members of the same subcultural background.

What was the dominant intellectual perspective in psychiatry in the 19th century throughout Europe and the United States?

Biological psychiatry.

What is circumstantiality?

It is a patient's discussion of unnecessary details and inappropriate thoughts before communicating a central idea. The patient should ultimately be able to reach the key point of the discussion.

Inability of the patient to reach the central point of a discussion even with sufficient time is called tangentiality.

What symptoms are associated with a dissociative phenomenon?

Derealization, depersonalization, dissociative amnesia, and fugue.

What is dissociation?

It is a splitting away of thoughts, feelings, or behaviors from conscious awareness.

What is the least clinically significant form of disorientation?

Disorientation to day or date. (It is so common that it happens in 60% of normal people.)

What should be accomplished during the initial assessment for psychodynamic psychotherapy?

An initial treatment plan, a mental-status assessment, a descriptive psychiatric diagnosis, and an initial psychodynamic formulation.

What is channeling?

Channeling is a meditative or trancelike state with the purpose of conveying messages from a spiritual guide. Channeling is often introduced as a culturally mediated, specific response to distress. It is considered a nonpathologic form of dissociation.

What is the serotonin syndrome?

It is the cluster of symptoms of restlessness, myoclonus, hyperreflexia, diaphoresis, shivering, tremor, and confusion, which usually follows the use of a monoamine oxidase inhibitor too soon after the failure of a tricyclic antidepressant (TCA) or selective serotonin reuptake inhibitor (SSRI), such that inadequate time was allowed to completely eliminate the TCA or SSRI from the body.

What is compulsion?

Repetitive, stereotyped behavior in which the patient recognizes the irrationality of the behavior.

What is Capgras syndrome?

The belief that an impostor has replaced a significant other (usually a family member).

What is Ganser syndrome?

The production of approximate answers (*vorbeireden*) to questions. This may be a manifestation of malingering, a state of confusion, or a disinhibition syndrome.

The term vorbeireden, circumlocution and failure to reach the central idea of a discussion, is not now popularly used in the psychiatric literature. Vorbeireden was sometimes used as an equivalent term to tangentiality.

What is alexithymia?

Difficulty in recognizing and describing one's emotions.

Is hallucination a part of the content of thought (COT)?

No. Inclusion of hallucination in COT is a popular mistake. Hallucination is a false sensory perception.

Between which two editions of the *Diagnostic and Statistical Manual of Mental Disorders* (DSM) did the diagnostic principle and approach to psychiatric illness undergo a major revision?

From DSM-II to DSM-III, in which a new medical model, with an evidence-based, research-driven approach replaced the psychodynamic theory-dominated model.

How is genuine auditory hallucination differentiated from malingering?

Thorough and prolonged examination and observation, plus good collateral information, may be the best way to differentiate the two. Reported characteristics of malingered auditory hallucination include the lack of a strategy to diminish the hallucinated voices, and reported use of stilted language by the voices (e.g., "Go commit a sex offense").

CHAPTER 7 Cognitive Disorders

Damage in which brain region is most likely to result in impaired social judgment?

Orbitofrontal area.

How does dementia with Lewy bodies differentiate from dementia of Alzheimer type?

Dementia with Lewy bodies is the second most common cause of dementia.

Typical symptoms are: More rapid decline in cognitive impairment; visual hallucinations; rapid eye movement (REM) behavior sleep disorder; and early extrapyramidal signs, very sensitive to typical neuroleptics.

Pathology: Lewy bodies in the cerebral cortex and basal ganglia are stained by α-synuclein antibodies.

What are chromosomal locations for Alzheimer disease–related mutations?

Chromosome 1: Presenilin 2, presents in <1% cases with onset at age 50 to 60 years.

Chromosome 14: Presenilin 1, presents in 1% to 5% cases with onset between age 30 and 50 years.

Chromosome 19: Apolipoprotein E (APO E), presents in 50% to 60% cases with age at onset 60 and older.

Chromosome 21: Amyloid precursor protein (APP) and β-amyloid, presents in <1% cases with age at onset of 40 to 50 years.

APP and *PS* genes are obligate factors, while APO E gene is a risk factor.

What remedies are available for the treatment of Alzheimer disease? What treatments are proposed and under investigation?

Cholinesterase inhibitors: Donepezil (Aricept), rivastigmine (Exelon), galanthamine (Razadyne).

N-methyl-D-aspartate (NMDA) antagonist: Memantine (Namenda).

Nonsteroidal anti-inflammatory drugs, estrogen replacement, and cholesterol-lowering medications were proposed for preventive treatment, but none proved effective in controlled studies.

Aβ vaccinations, γ secretase inhibitors, and stem cell implantation are experimental therapies under investigation.

What are risk factors for Alzheimer disease?

Age.

Family history.

APO E-4 gene, mutation in presenilin gene, and amyloid peptide precursor gene.

Mild to moderate risk factors: Female gender, head trauma, myocardial infarction, low education level.

What are the clinical manifestations of multi-infarct dementia?

Stepwise progression of deficits.

Pseudobulbar palsy.

Focal sensorimotor abnormalities.

What are the frontal lobe syndromes?

A variety of psychiatric symptoms that result from lesions in a frontal lobe.

Orbitofrontal syndrome: Disinhibition; impulsiveness; behaviors that are profane, irascible, and irresponsible.

Medial frontal syndrome: Apathy.

Left frontal syndrome: Depression.

Right frontal syndrome: Mania.

What are the neuroimaging findings in Alzheimer disease?

Neuroimaging methods do not yet have a clear role in the diagnosis of Alzheimer disease. Reported findings include:

Hypometabolism.

Atrophy in the frontal, parietal, and temporal lobes.

What are the pathologic characteristics of Pick disease?

Prominent frontotemporal atrophy.

Neuron cell inclusions: Clustered cytoskeletal elements.

Early personality and behavioral changes.

Other cognitive functions are relatively preserved.

What are the relative risk of Alzheimer disease referable to the *APO E-4* gene?

Apolipoprotein carries cholesterol and binds amyloid.

The *APO* gene is carried on chromosome 19. There are three alleles of the *APO* gene: *APO-E2, -E3,* and *-E4*.

The number of *APO-E4* gene copies is associated with the risk of Alzheimer disease. The relative risk is 1.0 (equivalent to that of the general population) for those with zero copies, 2.8 for one copy, and 8.1 for two copies.

What are the signs of normal aging?

Symptoms: Decreased muscle strength; loss of vibratory sensation; impaired balance; mild cognitive decline such as decreased attention span, slow acquisition of new information, difficulty in remembering names and recent events.

Slow electroencephalographic (EEG) background (<8 Hz).

Cerebral cortex atrophy. Brain weight decreases to about 85% of that of a normal adult.

Granulovacuolar degeneration, amyloid neuritic plaques, neurofibrillary tangles, loss of large cortical neurons.

No significant impairment in: Vocabulary, language, general information.

What disorder in early life has pathologic changes similar to those of Alzheimer disease?

Down syndrome.

Both Alzheimer disease and Down syndrome are associated with defects in chromosome 21.

Persons with Down syndrome who survive into early adulthood may present with histopathologic changes that are typical in Alzheimer disease (senile plaques and neurofibrillary tangles).

There is also a clear familial association of Alzheimer disease with Down syndrome.

What EEG features may appear in delirium?

Generalized slow wave (theta and delta) activity;

Sometimes focal areas of hyperactivity.

What is delirium?

Disturbance of consciousness.

Changes in attention, memory, orientation, language function, perception (hallucinations), behavior (agitation, wondering), and affect (labile mood).

Delirium usually develops over a short period and tends to fluctuate during the course of the day.

What is perseveration?

A disturbance in form of thought.

Often associated with cognitive disorders.

The patient exhibits a persisting response to a previous stimulus even after a new stimulus has been presented.

What is the most frequent cause of dementia in the United States?

Alzheimer disease.

What is the typical clinical presentation of frontotemporal dementia?

Early onset with a rapid decline. Mean age of onset of 53 years.

Disinhibition and Klüver-Bucy symptoms.

Early language disturbance, aphasia.

Memory impairment is less prominent in early stages.

Visual-spatial skills are relatively preserved.

The prototype is Pick disease.

What is the most significant risk factor for primary intracerebral hemorrhage?

Hypertension.

What is transient global amnesia?

Acute memory loss.

Tends to occur in middle-aged or elderly patients.

Primarily affects short-term memory, and typically lasts for hours.

Patients usually appear agitated, perplexed, and repeatedly inquire about their whereabouts, the time, and the nature of what they are experiencing.

Knowledge of personal identity is preserved, as are remote memories and perception.

The patient's obvious concern about the condition distinguishes transient global amnesia from other organically based amnestic syndromes and psychogenic amnesia.

What magnetic resonance imaging (MRI) finding is characteristic of multi-infarct dementia?

Multiple areas of increased T2-weighted density in the periventricular area.

What pathologic changes occur in frontotemporal dementia?

Prominent atrophy in frontal and temporal lobes.

Relatively normal parietal lobe.

Pick bodies: Argentophilic (silver-staining), intracytoplasmic.

Nonspecific neuronal loss.

Tau protein inclusion bodies.

About 10% of cases have mutation in the tau gene on chromosome 17.

Which type of memory do the hippocampus and parahippocampal gyrus mediate?

Declarative memory.

What tests should be considered in evaluating dementia?

Routine tests: Complete blood cell count, thyroid function, vitamin B12, homocysteine.

Consider if clinically indicated: Venereal Disease Research Laboratory, Lyme titer, human immunodeficiency virus.

Computed tomography and MRI are not required but are recommended by expert consensus.

EEG to rule out Creutzfeldt-Jakob disease and pseudodementia.

Lumbar puncture to rule out hydrocephalus, infectious diseases, cancer.

Psychometric testing is available to differentiate depression from dementia, and assess mental competence.

CHAPTER 8 Substance-Related Disorders

What does the motivational enhancement therapy (MET) model for addiction treatment emphasize?

The role of ambivalence in the process of change.

Which substance causes long-term inhibition of new serotonin synthesis and a decrease in serotonin terminal density?

Methylenedioxymethamphetamine (MDMA).

What is the unique feature for the diagnosis of polysubstance dependence?

A patient must meet dependency criteria for substances as a group, but not for any particular substance.

It is *not* that they meet criteria for dependency for more than one or two substance(s), or one dependency substance along with one or two abusing substance(s).

What role does levomethadyl acetate hydrochloride (LAAM) play in the management of opioid dependence?

The elimination of the need to take home doses.

Which area of the brain is most associated with the reward effects of cocaine?

Nucleus accumbens.

What are the purposes of pharmacologic treatment for alcoholism, and what agents are used to achieve them?

To reduce craving: Opioid antagonists (naltrexone, nalmefene), acamprosate, along with selective serotonin reuptake inhibitors (fluoxetine, citalopram), lithium, bromocriptine.

Withdrawal: Benzodiazepines (or barbiturates if benzodiazepines are not available).

Adverse conditioning: Disulfiram.

What is the characteristic electrophysiologic finding in alcoholic neuropathy?

Attenuated sensory and motor amplitudes.

What abnormalities in hepatic function tests are most likely to be associated with chronic alcohol abuse?

1. The γ-glutamyl transferase level is elevated in 80% of patients.
2. Serum glutamic oxaloacetic-transaminase (SGOT) and serum glutamic-pyruvic transaminase (SGPT) are both elevated, but SGOT is higher than SGPT.
3. Mean corpuscular volume is increased in 60% of patients.

What is idiosyncratic alcohol intoxication?

It is a severe behavioral syndrome that develops rapidly after a person consumes a small amount of alcohol that would have minimal behavioral effects on most people.

The patient can be confused and disoriented, and can have illusions, transitory delusions, and visual hallucinations, as well as displaying labile affect, slurred speech, and intoxicated behavior, with greatly increased psychomotor activity and impulsive, aggressive behavior that may be dangerous. The serum alcohol level is usually low (e.g., under 50 ng/dL).

This syndrome usually occurs in persons with high levels of anxiety or of advancing age, or with sedative-hypnotic drug use and a feeling of fatigue. The behavior tends to be atypical. This diagnosis is still debatable, but is important in the forensic arena.

Which subtype of anxiety disorder is most commonly associated with alcohol-related disorder?

Panic disorder.

What psychotic symptoms may present with alcohol withdrawal? What treatment is indicated?

Alcohol withdrawal may typically present with transient visual, tactile, or auditory hallucinations.

First-line treatment is a benzodiazepine. Low-dose, short treatment with antipsychotic agents may be needed.

What medication decreases the incidence of relapse in alcohol-dependent patients?

Naltrexone, but not disulfiram.

What are the mechanisms of action of disulfiram in reducing alcohol intake?

Disulfiram inhibits the alcohol-degrading enzyme acetaldehyde dehydrogenase, and therefore raises acetaldehyde levels in the blood and tissues. It also inhibits dopamine *β*-hydroxylase.

Its clinical effects last for up to 2 weeks after the last dose.

What are some characteristics of women with alcoholism?

Women with alcoholism are more likely to have onset at a later age, to have mood disorders, and to use other drugs.

What research data support the concept of hereditary factors in alcoholism?

The presence of hereditary factors for alcoholism were found in studies of adopted siblings. The famous Danish adoption studies of familial determinants of alcoholism demonstrated that biologic sons of alcoholic individuals were at higher risk of alcoholism than were biologic sons of nonalcoholic individuals.

What is the mission of Alcoholics Anonymous (Al-Anon)?

To help relatives cope with an alcoholic's drinking problem.

What drugs could be used to treat a patient who is in alcohol withdrawal who also has impaired liver function?

Oxazepam (Serax), lorazepam (Ativan), and temazepam (Restoril), because they do not have intermediate metabolic by-products that require further metabolism by the liver.

TOL—Tolerated by Our Liver.

What is the CAGE questionnaire?

A questionnaire used to screen patients for alcoholism. Its components have the meanings provided below:

*C*ut: Have you ever felt you should cut down on your drinking?

*A*nnoyed: Have people annoyed you by criticizing your drinking?

*G*uilt: Have you ever felt guilty about your drinking?

*E*ye-opener: Have you ever had a drink first thing in the morning to steady your nerves or to get rid of a hangover?

What is delirium tremens (DT)?

A severe alcohol withdrawal syndrome. It constitutes a medical emergency, and if untreated has a high mortality rate (20%).

DT usually occurs within 1 week after cessation of drinking. It has all the features of delirium. Other symptoms include:

1. Autonomic hyperactivity: Tachycardia, diaphoresis, fever, anxiety, insomnia, and hypertension.
2. A coarse tremor is common.
3. Seizures may occur early in the course of DT.

What is the substance most commonly abused by adolescents?

Alcohol.

The substance most commonly abused by the general population is nicotine.

What is the treatment for Wernicke syndrome?

<u>Give intravenous (IV) thiamine first!</u> Giving glucose without first replenishing thiamine may exhaust the body's remaining thiamine and worsen the patient's condition.

What is Wernicke-Korsakoff syndrome?

A persisting, alcohol-induced amnestic disorder.

Wernicke syndrome (also called alcoholic encephalopathy) is a condition of <u>acute onset</u> and is completely reversible.

Korsakoff syndrome is chronic, and only 20% of patients may recover.

Symptoms of Wernicke syndrome are:

- Ataxia.
- Confusion.
- Ophthalmoplegia (horizontal nystagmus, paralysis of the abducens, disconjugate eye movements, and gaze palsy).

Pathophysiology: Thiamine deficiency.

Horizontal nystagmus may also appear in phencyclidine intoxication, opioid withdrawal, and eighth cranial nerve impairment.

What are the maximum lengths of time for which cocaine metabolites and alcohol can be detected?

Cocaine metabolites: 2 to 4 days.

Alcohol: 7 to 12 hours.

What symptoms are related to cocaine withdrawal?

Hypersomnolence, dysphoria, mood irritability.

What beverage has the highest concentration of caffeine?

Concentrations of caffeine in the following beverages are in the order shown, from highest to lowest:

Dark chocolate.

Brewed coffee.

Instant coffee.

Tea (leaf or bagged).

Caffeinated soda.

What are the clinical features of cocaine intoxication?

1. Mental: Euphoria, hypervigilance, agitation or psychomotor retardation, hallucinations.

2. Cardiac: Tachycardia, bradycardia, high or low blood pressure, arrhythmia.
3. Other: Pupillary dilation, perspiration or chills, nausea, or vomiting.

Pupillary dilation: Cocaine, Opioid withdrawal, Lysergic acid diethylamide (LSD), Amphetamine intoxication. (Drink COLA, dilate pupils.)

How does cocaine work in the central nervous system?

Cocaine is a competitive blocker of the dopamine transporter. It inhibits dopamine reuptake and increases activation of dopaminergic pathways. It is sometimes called a dopamine agonist.

What is the medical complication commonly associated with cocaine abuse?

Myocardial infarction.

When does cocaine withdrawal occur?

Cocaine withdrawal occurs within hours to days after heavy cocaine use. It is characterized by dysphoria, increased appetite, fatigue, psychomotor retardation or agitation, and sleep abnormalities (dreams, insomnia, or hypersomnia).

Vivid, unpleasant dreams occur upon withdrawal from cocaine or amphetamine.

What are the clinical features of LSD intoxication?

1. Behavioral changes: Fear, anxiety, paranoid ideation, impaired judgment.
2. Perceptual changes: Perceptual changes in full wakefulness, depersonalization, derealization, illusions/hallucinations, and synesthesias.
3. Other: Pupillary dilation.

Synesthesia: A sensation or hallucination caused by another type of sensation.

Pupillary dilation: Cocaine, Opioid withdrawal, Lysergic acid diethylamide (LSD), Amphetamine intoxication. (Drink COLA, dilate pupils.)

What is the mechanism of action of LSD?

LSD is a partial agonist at postsynaptic serotonin receptors.

What is the most popular addictive substance in the United States?

The most popular addictive substance is nicotine.

Among all the abused substances, nicotine addiction contributes most to premature death and disability, and is associated with the highest annual mortality.

What pharmacologic treatment is available for nicotine dependence?

Bupropion (Zyban).

Varenicline (Chantix).

What are common opioid receptor ligands of the opioids?

Agonist: Methadone.

Antagonist: Naltrexone, naloxone, and nalmefene.

Agonist–antagonist (or partial agonist): Buprenorphine.

Naloxone and nalmefene: Rapid onset, IV use.

Naltrexone: Slower onset. Used in preventing relapse of alcoholism.

What are the mechanisms of action of opioids?

Opioids specifically bind μ, κ, δ, and probably other types of opioid receptors.

Opioids also have significant effects on the dopaminergic and noradrenergic systems.

Propranolol can potentiate opioid withdrawal symptoms.

Opium: *The dried, condensed juice of a poppy,* Papaver somniferum.

Opiate: "From opium." Extracts or derivatives of opium.

Opioid: "Opiumlike." Includes opiates (alkaloids; e.g., morphine) and endogenous opioids (peptides; e.g., endorphin). "Opioid" is more inclusive and is the preferred term.

What are the symptoms of opioid intoxication and withdrawal, and how are these conditions treated?

1. Opioid withdrawal symptoms are disorientation, confusion, dysphoric mood, vertical nystagmus, increased muscle tone, mildly enlarged pupils, increased blood pressure and heart rate, marked diaphoresis, piloerection, lacrimation (or rhinorrhea), salivation, nausea or vomiting, diarrhea, yawning, fever, and insomnia.
2. Opioid intoxication symptoms are pupillary constriction with drowsiness or coma, slurred speech, impairment of attention or memory, and pulmonary edema from central respiratory inhibition.

The pupils can be dilated from a severe opioid overdose, as a result of anoxia.

3. Treatment of withdrawal consists of giving clonidine or methadone.

4. Treatment of intoxication consists of giving naloxone at 0.4 mg IV for respiratory depression or stupor.

What should be done first to an opioid-intoxicated patient in the emergency room setting?

Ensure airway support and adequate ventilation. (Check the ABCs first!)

What is used to evaluate residual physical dependence in an opioid-dependent patient?

Naloxone.

What are the clinical features of phencyclidine (PCP) intoxication?

1. Neurologic: Vertical or horizontal nystagmus, numbness, ataxia, dysarthria, muscle rigidity.
2. Autonomic: Hypertension, increased bronchial and salivary secretions.
3. Mental: Hyperacusis, labile affect, agitation and aggressiveness.

PCP binds to the N-methyl-D-aspartate subtype of glutamate receptors.

Intoxication with what substance has the cluster of symptoms of ataxia, nystagmus, muscular rigidity, normal or small pupils, and stupor?

PCP.

What is the medical complication commonly associated with PCP abuse?

Rhabdomyolysis.

According to the DSM-IV-TR what are the differences between the diagnostic criteria for substance abuse and dependence?

In both diagnoses, the condition must have persisted for a 12-month period.

Abuse consists of any of the following: Continued substance use despite interpersonal problems; failure to fulfill obligations, potential physical harm caused by substance use, and recurrent substance-related legal problems; social/occupational dysfunction.

Dependence consists of three of the following: Tolerance, withdrawal, use of increasing amounts of a substance, an unsuccessful attempt at cessation, spending considerable time using a substance, dysfunction, and continuing use despite problems.

When criteria for both abuse and dependence are met, the diagnosis is dependence.

What criteria differentiate substance dependence from substance abuse?

Tolerance and withdrawal, use of a substance in larger amounts and/or for longer periods than desired, failure to reduce the use of a substance, considerable time spent using the substance.

What are the symptoms of intoxication with *Cannabis sativa*?

Conjunctival injection, increased appetite, dry mouth, and tachycardia with behavioral changes.

What is the average half-life of marijuana (tetrahydrocannabinol metabolites) in the human body?

From 2 to 7 weeks.

For what is the pentobarbital challenge test used?

Estimating the starting dose for barbiturate detoxification.

What psychopharmacologic agents are indicated to treat PCP intoxication?

Antipsychotic agents and benzodiazepines.

What are the clinical features of amphetamine abuse/dependence?

Chronic abuse of amphetamines may cause intracerebral vasculitis and hemorrhage.

Amphetamine withdrawal may cause vivid, unpleasant dreams.

Vivid, unpleasant dreams occur upon withdrawal from cocaine or amphetamine.

Cook and dream! (Coc-Am-Dream.)

What are the risk factors for completed suicide in persons who have a chemical dependency problem?

DEAD:

D: Drug (history of drug overdose).

E: Ethanol (use of alcohol concurrently with drugs).

A: Abrupt (abrupt decision to commit suicide).

D: Desperate (recent personal loss).

Withdrawal from what substance can cause insomnia, extreme anxiety and tremulousness, and grand mal seizures?

Sedating agents such as diazepam, alcohol, and barbiturates.

CHAPTER 9 Psychotic Disorders, Mood Disorders, and Anxiety Disorders

How common are the anxiety disorders?

The most prevalent psychiatric disorders.

Lifetime prevalence of any anxiety: 25%.

Lifetime prevalence of social phobia and simple phobia is higher than that of panic disorder, agoraphobia, and generalized anxiety disorder.

More likely to have anxiety disorders: Women; first-degree relatives of patients with anxiety disorders.

Less likely to have anxiety disorders: Men; higher socioeconomic status.

By what mechanisms is S-adenosyl methionine (SAMe) and methylfolate applied in the treatment of depression?

Abnormalities in one carbon cycle metabolism are associated with clinical depression, presumably due to deficiency in monoamine neurotransmitters.

SAMe is the major donor of methyl groups in the synthesis of monoamine neurotransmitters, including serotonin, norepinephrine, and dopamine.

Methylfolate is an important element in replenishing SAMe.

Folic acid is the precursor of methylfolate.

The conversion of folic acid to methylfolate relies on an enzyme, 5,10-methylene tetrahydrofolate reductase (MTHFR).

MTHFR polymorphism may decrease the availability of methylfolate.

Oral methylfolate and SAMe may help replenish SAMe, and have been suggested as supplements for treatment of depression.

How is uncomplicated, or "normal," bereavement differentiated from major depressive disorder?

Symptoms that indicate complication of major depression:

Suicidal ideation;

Guilt;

Psychomotor retardation;

Hallucination;

Preoccupation with worthlessness;

Symptoms lasting longer than 2 months.

Uncomplicated bereavement may present with extreme sadness, crying spells, and anger toward God; however, it does not present with the symptoms mentioned above.

How is substance-induced mood disorder diagnosed?

Mood symptoms must appear after the onset of substance use;

Mood symptoms may appear during intoxication or withdrawal.

Mood symptoms must exceed those usually associated with intoxication or withdrawal, and must be severe enough to warrant clinical attention for a separate diagnosis.

In patients with anxiety disorders, what are the risk factors that indicate the possibility of an organic etiology?

Onset after age 40.

Lack of familial history.

Lack of triggering events.

Lack of avoidance behavior.

Poor response to anxiolytic agents.

Is "anxiety neurosis" a form of anxiety disorder?

Anxiety neurosis is a term coined by Sigmund Freud.

According to Freud, an escalation in sexual tension leads to an increase in libido and desire for intercourse. When a sexual outlet is unavailable, the unreleased tension produces neurosis.

The symptoms described by Freud are similar to those for panic disorder as defined in DSM-IV-TR.

Freud held that libidinal blockage related to heightened anxiety is the biological basis of several neuroses including neurasthesia, hypochondriasis, and anxiety neuroses.

Is mitral valve prolapse a contributing factor to panic disorder?

Mitral valve prolapse was believed to be associated with panic disorder, and historically has raised great research interest.

However, extensive research has found mitral valve prolapse to be unrelated to panic disorder.

What are clinical features of posttraumatic stress disorder (PTSD)?

Re-experiencing of the traumatic event;

Increased arousal;

Avoidance of stimuli;

Numbing of general responsiveness;

Persistence of symptoms for longer than 1 month.

What are common comorbid conditions in bipolar disorder?

Substance abuse.

Anxiety disorders.

Attention-deficit/hyperactivity disorder.

What are prodromal and residual symptoms of schizophrenia?

Social isolation;

Impairment of functioning;

Peculiar behavior;

Impaired personal hygiene;

Blunted or inappropriate affect;

Abnormal speech;

Odd beliefs.

What are Schneiderian First Rank Symptoms and what is their role in diagnosis of schizophrenia?

A group of positive symptoms described by German psychiatrist Kurt Schneider, and believed to be specific for schizophrenia.

Including audible thoughts, voices heard arguing, voices heard commenting on one's actions, thought withdrawal, thought broadcast, imposed feelings, imposed impulses, and delusional perception. All are positive symptoms.

Schneider believed the diagnosis of schizophrenia can be made with non–first rank symptoms.

The diagnostic reliability of first rank symptoms has been questioned, and the majority of mental health professionals do not use them as diagnostic aids.

What are the common sequelae experienced by victims of rape?

Shame;

PTSD symptoms;

Sexual difficulties.

What are the comorbid conditions commonly seen with anxiety disorders?

The majority of patients with panic disorder and/or agoraphobia have other psychiatric disorders.

Common comorbid disorders are: Major depressive disorder; another anxiety disorder; hypochondriasis; personality disorders; substance-related disorders.

What are the factors associated with a good prognosis in schizophrenia?

Good premorbid functioning;

Little prodrome;

Late age of onset;

Acute onset of disease;

Positive symptoms;

Confusion or perplexity at the height of the psychotic episode;

Female gender;

Absence of a family history of psychotic illness.

What are the negative symptoms in schizophrenia?

Flat affect.

Abulia (lack of impulses to act and think, indifference).

Acathexis (lack of appropriate emotional response).

Alogia (poverty of speech).

Avolition (lack of desire, motivation, and persistence).

What are the neurophysiologic mechanisms of anxiety disorders?

Serotoninergic systems: Modulators of γ-aminobutyric acid (GABA) and noradrenergic systems.

Noradrenergic system: Stimulation of the locus ceruleus, where noradrenergic neurons are located, may induce panic attacks.

GABA system: Widely distributed with highest density in the limbic system. Binding with benzodiazepines reduces anxiety.

What brain image changes may present in major depressive disorder?

Enlarged ventricles.

Decreased volumes of the frontal lobes, the hippocampus, and the basal ganglia.

Hypofrontality, or decreased metabolic activity in the frontal cortex; this may be reversed by positive response to antidepressant treatment.

Global reduction in cerebral blood flow.

What are "panicogens"?

Panicogens are anxiety-inducing substances, usually used in research to create paniclike reactions.

Commonly used panicogens include: Carbon dioxide, sodium lactate, bicarbonate, yohimbine, 1-(meta-chlorophenyl)piperazine (mCPP), flumazenil, cholecystokinin, caffeine, isoproterenol.

What is dementia praecox?

The former name for schizophrenia;

Emil Kraepelin was the first author to describe the disease, calling it dementia praecox;

It literally means "early onset dementia";

Eugen Bleuler renamed it as schizophrenia.

What is neurosis?

The term was originally coined by Scottish physician William Cullen and literally means "nervous disease."

Sigmund Freud defined neurosis as symptoms presenting when the ego's efforts to resolve emotional conflicts between the id and superego using defense mechanisms fail.

What is schizophrenia's pattern of inheritance?

Monozygotic: 45% to 50% concordance.

Dizygotic: 10% to 15% concordance.

Risk for children or siblings of a schizophrenic patient: 10%.

What is the age of onset for schizophrenia?

Male: 18 to 25 years.

Female: 26 to 45 years.

What is the average age of onset for unipolar depression?

Twenty-nine years.

What is the average lifetime number of episodes for unipolar depression?

Four.

What medical conditions are commonly associated with anxiety symptoms?

Drug/substance: Cocaine, caffeine, thyroid hormones, theophylline, corticosteroids, sympathomimetics. Withdrawal from alcohol, narcotics, benzodiazepines.

Endocrine: Hyperthyroidism, hyperparathyroidism, pheochromocytoma.

Cardiovascular: Arrhythmias, mitral valve prolapse (controversial).

Pulmonary: Pulmonary embolism, chronic obstructive pulmonary disease.

What is the lifetime rate of completed suicide in bipolar disorder?

Up to 15%.

What neuronal circuits are believed to be relevant to anxiety disorders?	Brainstem: Noradrenergic neurons of the locus ceruleus, serotonergic neurons of the median raphe nucleus. Temporal lobes, particularly the hippocampus: Cortical atrophy, cerebral blood flow dysregulation. Amygdala, midbrain, and hypothalamus: Local inhibition of GABAergic transmission.
What sleep abnormalities are associated with major depressive disorder?	Shortened rapid-eye-movement (REM) sleep latency. Decreased non-REM sleep. Increased REM density. Reduced total sleep time. Decreased stage IV sleep; Increased awakening during the second half of the night.
What types of hallucinations may occur in delusional disorder?	Hallucinations are rare in delusional disorder; Tactile and olfactory hallucinations may occur in delusional disorder, and are usually associated with the delusional theme.
What was the important insight that made Emil Kraepelin a towering figure in the history of psychiatry?	That major mental illnesses have different courses and outcomes; Kraepelin believed that dementia praecox follows a course of declining cognition, but that manic depressive disorder does not.

CHAPTER 10

Personality Disorders and Other Clinical Conditions

What diagnoses are categorized as somatoform disorders?

The following seven diagnoses are offered in DSM-IV under the category of somatoform disorders:

1. Somatization disorder (also known as Briquet syndrome).
2. Conversion disorder.
3. Hypochondriasis.
4. Pain disorder.
5. Body dysmorphic disorder.
6. Undifferentiated somatoform disorder.
7. Somatoform disorder not otherwise specified.

What is conversion disorder?

Conversion disorder consists of neurologic symptoms that cannot be explained by a known medical disorder. The symptoms are not intentionally produced, and not limited to pain or sexual dysfunction. Psychological factors are judged to be associated with the symptoms.

What are the differential diagnosis for conversion disorder?

If non-neurologic symptoms are present, somatization disorder should be considered the proper diagnosis.

If symptoms are intentionally produced, factitious disorder or malingering should be considered.

If only pain or sexual dysfunction is present, pain or sexual disorders should be considered.

What medical conditions have presentations similar to that of somatization disorder?

Many medical conditions have presentations similar to that of somatization disorder. Common ones include:

Multiple sclerosis.

Acute intermittent porphyria.

Systemic lupus erythematosus.

Fibromyositis.

Endocrine disorders.

Chronic infections.

What is the most common electrolyte imbalance seen in eating disorders?

Hypokalemia.

When cardiac disturbance (anxiety, palpitation) are suspected, check the patient's serum potassium concentration.

What are the major complications of anorexia nervosa?

General: *Cachexia, edema,* lanugo, electrolyte imbalance, decreased body temperature.

Mental: Depression.

Cardiac: Loss of cardiac muscle, change in heart rate.

Gastrointestinal: Digestive dysfunction.

Sexual: Amenorrhea.

Hematologic: Leukopenia.

Musculoskeletal: Osteoporosis, dental erosion.

What would the laboratory workup show in an adolescent girl with anorexia nervosa?

Low hematocrit, high cortisol, and high blood urea nitrogen concentration.

In comparison to patients with anorexia nervosa, what is characteristic in patients with involuntary starvation?

A reduced activity level.

Patients with eating disorders usually have an increased activity level.

What pharmacologic treatment is used for eating disorders?

Antidepressants, with selective serotonin reuptake inhibitors (SSRIs) being the agents of first choice.

Tricyclic antidepressants such as imipramine and desipramine, as well as monoamine oxidase inhibitors, are helpful, but these are not the first choice if SSRIs are available.

Mirtazapine and venlafaxine are not well studied in eating disorders.

Bupropion is contraindicated in eating disorders.

A patient complains of snoring at night, and being irritable and drowsy during the daytime. What diagnostic test should be ordered?

Polysomnography.

What are the respiratory manifestations of sleep apnea?

Central: Lack of inspiratory effort.

Obstructive: Increased inspiratory effort.

What are clinical features of narcolepsy?

Episodes of sudden onset of sleep occurring daily for more than 3 months, and that present with one or both of the following features:

1. Cataplexy (sudden loss of muscle tone, often precipitated by strong emotion), followed by the patient's entry into rapid-eye-movement (REM) sleep within a few minutes after falling asleep;
2. Repeated intrusions of REM sleep into the transition between sleep and wakefulness (as manifested by hypnopompic or hypnagogic hallucinations or sleep paralysis).

What is the first choice in initial treatment for primary insomnia?

Sleep hygiene (restricting the use of the bed to sleep only).

What observations are characteristic during REM sleep?

Tachycardia.

Penile tumescence.

Atonia.

Rapid eye movements.

Dreaming.

Relatively low-voltage mixed-frequency waves in the electroencephalogram.

What characteristics are usually reported of patients with obstructive sleep apnea?

Obesity.

Frequent daytime napping.

Snoring at bedtime.

Early-morning awakening and inability to return to sleep are associated with what clinical conditions?

Depression.

Advanced sleep-phase syndrome.

Alcohol abuse.

Mania.

What is the most appropriate initial intervention for sleep apnea?

Continuous positive airway pressure (CPAP).

What are typical presentations of narcissistic personality disorder?

Arrogance.

Haughty behavior.

Belief by the subject that he or she is special.

Need for excessive admiration.

Envy of others.

Lack of empathy.

Sense of entitlement.

Tendency toward exploitation in interpersonal relationships.

Grandiosity; extreme sense of self-importance.

What clinical features might differentiate borderline personality disorder from histrionic personality disorder?

Both disorders are marked by labile affect, seductiveness, exaggerated anger, and volatile relationships.

Self-mutilation is frequent in patients with borderline personality disorder.

What is sleep terror syndrome?

A subtype of parasomnia.

It is characterized by recurrent episodes of abrupt awakening from sleep, usually during the first third of a major sleep episode, with a panicky scream, intense fear, and signs of autonomic arousal during each episode.

The patient is usually relatively unresponsive to the efforts of others to comfort them.

No detailed dream is recalled.

Sleep terror syndrome is more frequent in children than in adults.

What is the difference between sleep terror syndrome and nightmares?

In nightmare disorder, the details of dreams can be recalled. Awakening in this disorder usually occurs in the second half of the sleep period. However, in sleep terror syndrome, no detailed dream is recalled.

What are the most and least prevalent male sexuality disorders?

Most prevalent: Male erectile disorder.

Least prevalent: Male orgasmic disorder.

What is fetishism?

A condition in which an individual is sexually aroused by inanimate objects, such as undergarments or high-heeled shoes. Male persons with this disorder may be caught *stealing women's clothing.*

What is the main symptom of transvestic fetishism?	Cross-dressing.
Which sexual and gender identity disorder primarily involves homosexual individuals?	None. According to the American Psychiatric Association, homosexuality is a lifestyle rather than a pathologic phenomenon.
What is homophobia?	A persistently negative attitude toward or fear of homosexuality or homosexuals.
What is dyspareunia?	Recurrent or persistent genital pain associated with sexual intercourse. It may occur in either men or women, and can happen before or after intercourse. Both medical and psychologic conditions can contribute to its development.
What is the minimum time criterion for the diagnosis of paraphilia?	Six months.
What does the nocturnal penile tumescence monitoring test evaluate?	Erectile capacity.
What is *attaque de nervios*?	A culture-restricted syndrome among Latino persons from the Caribbean. It is marked by shouting, crying, trembling, anger, a sensation of heat in the chest and head, headache, verbal and physical aggression, insomnia, and despair. It includes no acute fear (as distinguished from panic attack). Persons with *attaque de nervios* may experience amnesia, but rapidly return to their usual functional state.

What is Couvade syndrome?	A culture-bound syndrome in which a father takes to his bed during or shortly after the birth of his child, as though he himself had given birth.
What is Amok?	A culture-bound syndrome found in Malayans. It appears as a dissociative episode with a violent outburst. Accompanying symptoms include persecutory delusions, automatism, and amnesia.

CHAPTER 11 Psychiatry and Law

How does one evaluate a patient's competency to give adequate informed consent?

Competency is declared by a court, not a physician.

Clinical assessment of capacity to make treatment decisions is sometimes called "competency evaluation," though this is technically incorrect.

Capacity can be global or task specific.

Evaluating the capacity to make treatment decisions requires the following information:

Factual understanding of the information.

Appreciation of the seriousness of the condition and consequences of accepting or rejecting treatment.

Ability to manipulate the information in a rational fashion and come to a decision logically.

Communication of a preference.

Under what circumstances can the requirement of informed consent be exempted?

Emergency situations when failure to provide treatment may result in serious damage.

The patient's waiver for decision making, which usually implies trust in someone else's judgment.

Therapeutic privilege. The physician has therapeutic privilege when the process of obtaining consent is judged harmful to the patient. This usually means not a complete exemption, but a deferred process.

If a psychiatrist who is a former employee of an institution wants to write articles for publication about his or her clinical cases while at the institution, what steps should the psychiatrist take?

The psychiatrist should keep a separate set of process notes, which are <u>his or her personal property rather than the property of the institution</u>.

Under what circumstance may a patient refuse treatment?

Competent individuals have a right to make their own treatment decisions, including refusal of treatment that others believe is in their best interest.

When a patient is deemed incapacitated and unable to make treatment decisions, an alternative decision maker should be sought.

Decisions on routine and ordinary care may be made by family members who know the patient well.

Decisions on extraordinary, invasive, or dangerous procedures should be made by a guardian.

Depending on state laws, some extraordinary treatments may require court authorization.

Allowing an incapacitated patient to continue making treatment decisions is unethical.

According to the American Psychiatric Association and the World Psychiatric Association, may a psychiatrist participate in the legal execution of a prisoner?

No. Both organizations consider this behavior to be unethical, and maintain that psychiatrists should not participate in executions.

What are professional boundaries?

The basic principle of boundary is that the physician is obligated to put the best interests of the patient ahead of the physician's interests. Any behavior that may favor the physician's interests over the patient's interests may cause boundary violations.

The nature of the action and the situation determine the boundary.

It is the physician's responsibility, not the patient's, to maintain appropriate boundaries.

What behaviors are commonly considered violation of boundary?

Sexual contact between a current patient and a physician of any specialty.

Sexual contact between a current or former patient and a psychiatrist.

Business dealings between doctor and patient.

Nonsexual social contact with a patient, unless it is unavoidable.

What are the general indications for seclusion and restraint of a patient?

Prevention of harm to the patient or others.

Use of seclusion and restraint as ongoing behavioral treatment and to decrease stimulation.

Seclusion and restraint <u>should not be used as a punishment</u> for violent or other undesired behaviors.

What are the requirements of the Patient Self-Determination Act for patients admitted to a hospital?

Patients must receive written or printed information advising them of their right:

To refuse treatment.

To ask for advance directives.

To designate a health care proxy.

What ethical principle provides the most appropriate basis for psychiatric intervention in the case of a mentally incompetent patient?

Beneficence.

What is fiduciary duty?

The responsibility of a physician to act in a patient's best interests.

What is HIPAA?

Health Insurance Portability and Accountability Act, a law enacted by the U.S. Congress in 1996.

HIPAA protects health insurance coverage for workers and their families when they change or lose their jobs.

HIPAA requires the establishment of national standards for electronic health care transactions, and encourages the use of electronic data interchange in the U.S. health care system.

HIPAA addresses the security and privacy of health data.

What is paternalism?

Paternalism is a philosophical principal that stems from the tradition that the family is a model for all organizations.

In medicine, paternalism implies that a physician is acting in the best interest of a patient whose own capacity for autonomous decision making is severely impaired.

What is required by the concept of informed consent?

Informed consent requires a thorough discussion with the patient of:

Indications for treatment.

The inability to predict the results of the treatment, and the possible risks and adverse effects of the treatment.

Alternative forms of treatment.

The risks of not having treatment.

To be able to give informed consent, a patient must have:

<u>Sufficient information</u> to understand the treatment.

To be <u>mentally competent</u> to make a voluntary choice.

What is the most important factor in determining the competency of a patient who refuses a recommended therapeutic procedure?	The patient's adequate understanding of the medical consequences of not undergoing the procedure.
What is the legal basis for most psychiatrists to prescribe a medication that is not approved by the U.S. Food and Drug Administration (FDA)?	The FDA regulates drug manufacturing and marketing, not medical practice. A physician should make treatment decisions based on all the available data, including but not limited to those supported by FDA. The physician is allowed to prescribe a medicine that to his or her best knowledge is probably effective for the patient's condition.
What should a patient be told when undergoing a psychiatric examination to determine suitability for a job?	The examination is not confidential. There is no therapeutic alliance with the psychiatrist giving the examination.
What should a psychiatrist assess when evaluating a patient's competency to make a will?	The psychiatrist should confirm that the patient understands: He or she is making a will. How the will distributes his or her property. The nature and extent of his or her property subject to distribution by the will. The persons who would normally be expected to benefit from the will.

What was the legal principle formulated after the case of Tarasoff versus the Board of Regents of the University of California?

The clinician has the responsibility:

To warn the intended victims of dangerous patients, and

To take steps to protect the intended victims.

When a patient who appears to lack the capacity to make treatment decisions refuses treatment, what should a physician do?

Evaluate the capacity for decision making.

If the patient is capable of decision making, follow the patient's preference.

If the patient is incapable of decision making, and if the treatment is ordinary and noninvasive (such as use of antidepressants and anxiolytics), look for an alternative decision maker, such as a family member, or use therapeutic privilege.

If the patient is incapable of decision making, and if the treatment is extraordinary and invasive (such as use of antipsychotics and electroconvulsive therapy), seek the formal guardian or obtain a court order.

CHAPTER 12 Consultation-Liaison Psychiatry

What is the mechanism of menopause?

It is the progressive insensitivity of the ovary to the effect of follicle-stimulating hormone (FSH).

What type of somatoform disorder has the best prognosis?

Conversion disorder.

What is a possible psychiatric comorbidity with a left prefrontal cerebrovascular accident patient?

Depression.

What is risk factor for the development of postpartum psychosis?

Maternal history of puerperal psychiatric illness.

A 23-year-old woman was referred to a psychiatrist by a plastic surgeon. She constantly complains that part of her face is swollen; however, the surgeon could not document her claim. What is the most likely diagnosis?

Body dysmorphic disorder.

What conditions may cause catatonia?

Conditions that may cause catatonia are:

Mania.

Neurologic disorders (e.g., encephalitis).

Depression.

Schizophrenia.

Ingestion of phencyclidine.

Other psychiatric conditions.

Electrolyte imbalances, such as hypocalcemia, do not cause catatonia.

What is the drug of choice for rapid tranquilization?

Haloperidol given intramuscularly.

If the patient is willing and able to take an oral drug, the choice would be equivocal. Recent research shows risperidone to be as effective as haloperidol and to have a comparably rapid onset of action and a better side-effect profile. Intramuscular ziprasidone and olanzepine are emerging new treatments.

What is the major concern in acetaminophen overdose?

Hepatotoxicity.

What are some important factors in evaluating chronic pain?

The patient's ethnic background may influence the symptoms.

Depression may present as chronic pain.

One third of patients respond to a placebo.

What medical conditions should be ruled out in patients with acute extreme anxiety?

Alcohol withdrawal.

Pulmonary embolism.

Use of sympathomimetic agents.

What is the most useful diagnostic tool for patients with suspected delirium?

The Mini-Mental Status Examination (MMSE).

What is the role of benzodiazepines in controlling delirium?

As a general rule, benzodiazepines should be avoided in cases of delirium. Benzodiazepines may cause increased confusion, disinhibition, falling, and behavioral problems.

What is the best agent for managing steroid-induced mania?

Usually, a low-dose antipsychotic agent, because of these drugs' rapid effect.

Benzodiazepines may cause more confusion.

Antidepressants and mood-stabilizing drugs take weeks to produce effects, and are therefore not used.

What characteristics are more likely in elderly than in young patients with medical surgical conditions?

<u>Delirium.</u>

Adverse reactions to <u>anticholinergic drugs.</u>

What is the most important risk factor for postpartum psychosis?

A history of puerperal psychiatric illness.

Age, complications of delivery, and multiparity are not risk factors for postpartum psychosis.

What are the essential responsibilities for a physician requesting a psychiatric consultation?

The physician should prepare the patient for the consultation and clearly state the reason for, urgency of, and expectations from the consultation.

What symptoms may acute intermittent porphyria present, and what test could be diagnostic for this condition?

The symptoms of acute intermittent porphyria include colicky abdominal pain with nausea and vomiting, psychosis (e.g., hallucinations), agitated depression, and polyneuropathy.

Acute intermittent porphyria has been estimated to be undiagnosed in 0.5% of psychiatric patients.

The clinical diagnostic test for the condition is the porphobilinogen test.

If a postsurgical patient reports inadequate pain relief after having intramuscular (IM) meperidine replaced by oral (PO) meperidine at the same dosage and frequency, what is likely to be the reason for this problem?

Meperidine PO has a lower analgesic potency than IM meperidine.

What is the earliest symptom of delirium?

Impaired attention. Mood fluctuation, agitation, insomnia, and psychosis may follow.

What is the neuropsychiatric presentation of HIV infection?

Memory impairment (dementia).

Pathologic slowing of information processing.

Dysgraphia.

Leg weakness.

Delirium.

Anxiety disorders.

	Adjustment disorders.
	Depressive disorders.
	Substance abuse.
What should be done for a terminally ill patient who is in the bargaining stage of reacting to his or her impending death?	Assure the patient that he or she will be given the best care regardless of the patient's behavior.
What should be done for a patient who is in denial of an untreatable illness?	Ensure that the patient has been informed about the illness and the treatment that can be given for it.
What is the most important principle in helping dying patients?	Preserve the patient's hope.
What is malingering?	The intentional production of false or grossly exaggerated physical or psychological symptoms, motivated by external incentives.
What psychiatric symptoms might be related to left-frontal-lobe damage?	Depression.
How do questions about suicide influence patients' suicidal behavior?	Questions about suicide do not influence the likelihood of a suicide attempt.
What is the most common mental disorder of elderly patients with acute and chronic medical conditions in primary-care settings?	Depression.

What is neurasthenia?

A term used to describe the condition currently known as chronic fatigue syndrome.

Neurasthenia is still a popular diagnosis in China.

In what malignant condition can the initial presentation be depression?

Carcinoma of the pancreas.

What agents may be used to prevent akathisia (anxiety, agitation, fidgeting, need to move constantly, and a strong sensation of being uncomfortable)?

β-blockers (treatment of choice).

Benzodiazepines.

Anticholinergic agents.

Amantadine.

Clonidine.

A patient had a head concussion 4 days before being brought to psychiatric attention. He was doing well until 2 hours ago, when his mental status began to change. What is the test of choice?

Magnetic resonance imaging is preferred to computed tomography. An imaging scan should be done before a spinal tap. Radiography of the skull or electroencephalography is not diagnostic.

What is the best psychiatric group-treatment strategy for patients with metastasized breast cancer?

Supportive expressive group therapy.

What is the best group-treatment strategy for patients at risk for AIDS?

Educational groups.

What psychiatric medication may exacerbate symptoms of psoriasis?	Lithium.
What medication is indicated for severe alcohol withdrawal?	A benzodiazepine.
How do antidepressants influence the seizure threshold?	Selective serotonin reuptake inhibitors may not influence the seizure threshold. Bupropion, tricyclic antidepressants, and tetracyclic antidepressants may lower the seizure threshold.
With what neuropsychiatric symptoms can digitalis toxicity present?	Depression. Manic-like behavior. Agitation. Visual abnormalities with scotoma, flickering halos, and objects appearing to have yellow-green borders.
What are typical symptoms of vitamin B_{12} deficiency?	Abnormal proprioception. Dysesthesia. Dementia. Macrocytic anemia.
When a patient in a medical unit develops dysarthria with a protruding tongue and torticollis, what medication should be suspected?	An antiemetic such as: Metoclopramide (Reglan). Promethazine (Phenergan).

Prochlorperazine (Compazine).

These medications are widely used in medical units. They have dopamine-antagonistic effects and may cause extrapyramidal side effects.

What is catatonia and how is it treated?

Catatonia is a cluster of symptoms that may present with:

Motor immobility (catalepsy or stupor).

Excessive motor activity.

Extreme negativism (rigid posture upon externally attempted movements).

Mutism.

Peculiarities of voluntary movement (bizarre postures).

Stereotyped movements.

Prominent mannerisms.

Prominent grimacing.

Echolalia.

Echopraxia.

The treatment of choice is a benzodiazepine. Lorazepam given intramuscularly has well-documented efficacy in catatonia.

Catatonia occurs most commonly in bipolar affective disorder (45% of cases) and neurologic disease (40% of cases), and much less often in schizophrenia (5% to 10% of cases).

What is postconcussional disorder?

After a head-trauma accident that causes significant cerebral concussion, the affected individual may display:

Difficulty in focusing attention or with memory.

Headache.

Vertigo or dizziness.

Irritability.

Emotional lability.

Depression.

Fatigue.

Disturbed sleep.

Changes in personality.

Apathy or lack of spontaneity.

These symptoms should last at least 3 months for a diagnosis of postconcussional disorder.

CHAPTER 13 Child Psychiatry

What are the clinical characteristic features of the Rett disorder?

Normal prenatal, perinatal, and psychomotor development through the first 5 months after birth.

Normal head circumference at birth.

Deceleration of head growth beginning in early childhood (5 to 48 months).

Loss of previously acquired purposeful hand skills and subsequent development of stereotyped hand movements (e.g., hand-wringing or hand-washing).

Loss of social engagement.

Poor coordination in gait or trunk movement.

Severe impairment of expressive and receptive language development.

Severe psychomotor retardation.

Children with Turner syndrome are most likely to manifest what sexual behavior during adulthood?

Heterosexuality.

What are the core features of the Prader-Willi syndrome?

Mental retardation.

Obesity.

Short stature.

Hypogonadism.

Hyperphagia.

Chromosome 15 deletion exists in 70% of cases.

How should one manage the school phobia associated with nonpsychotic separation anxiety in a preadolescent child?

Rapidly return the child to school.

Though proper support is helpful, parents should avoid rewarding undesired behavior.

What most significantly affects a child's psychological adjustment to the divorce of his or her parents?

The amount of parental conflict after the divorce.

What are the adverse effects of methylphenidate?

Emotional lability.

Weight loss.

Insomnia.

Decreasing tricyclic antidepressant concentration.

Rebound hyperactivity.

According to Erik Erikson, the developmental crisis most typical of normal middle age involves what?

Generativity versus stagnation.

What are the choices of pharmacologic treatment for attention-deficit/ hyperactivity disorder (ADHD)?

Psychostimulants: Methylphenidate (Ritalin, Methylin, Metadate, Concerta); dexmethylphenidate (Focalin); dextroamphetamine (Dexedrine, Dextrostat); and dextroamphetamine/amphetamine (Adderall).

Selective norepinephrine reuptake inhibitor: Atomoxetine (Strattera).

Central α-agonists: Guanfacine (Tenex); and clonidine (Catapres).

Antidepressants: Imipramine (Anafranil); bupropion (Wellbutrin); desipramine (Norpramin).

In the emergency room of a hospital, a young child holds his familiar blanket. As what does this blanket serve?

A transitional object.

What are the differences in the diagnostic criteria for a major depressive episode in children as compared to adults?

In children, the diagnostic criteria for a major depressive episode are the same as for adults, except that:

Mood change can present as irritable mood instead of depressed mood. Prepubertal children have more frequent episodes of irritable mood than do adult depressive patients.

Instead of significant weight loss, children with depression may present with failure to make expected weight gains.

What are the major fears of a $2^1/_2$-year-old child who is hospitalized?

Separation and abandonment.

What behavior differentiates conduct disorder from other behavior disorders in a prepubertal child?	Initiating fights. Bullying. Threatening or intimidating others. Physical cruelty to people and/or animals. Stealing. Forcing others to have sex. Arson and/or destruction of others' property. Breaking into others' houses or automobiles. Lying. Staying out at night before the age of 13 years. Running away from home. Truancy from school.
What characteristic of manic disorder is more likely in prepubertal children than in adult patients?	Irritability as opposed to euphoria.
What diagnosis comorbid with ADHD carries the worst prognosis?	Conduct disorder.
What factors must be ruled out in the diagnosis of enuresis?	Organic factors, such as urinary tract infections.

What is anaclitic depression?

Described by René Spitz.

Refers to children who become depressed and nonresponsive after prolonged separation from their mothers.

What is frequently seen in the members of an incestuous family?

Denial of sexual content of behavior.

What is hospitalism?

Described by René Spitz.

Refers to infants who waste away while in hospital.

Caused by multiple etiologies; however, the main cause was believed to be lack of social contact.

It was also found that this condition occurred less frequently in hospitals for indigents, where staff members hold the infants more often due to the lack of funding to afford equipment such as incubators.

What is most likely to be a manifestation of selective mutism in children?

Anxiety disorders.

What is the appropriate reaction to the parents of a 2-year-old child who has not begun to speak intelligibly?

Most children of this age can effectively make themselves understood.

Appropriate evaluation may be suggested.

What is the core feature of fragile X syndrome?

The triad of a long face, prominent ears, and macro-orchidism.

ADHD appears in 80% of patients.

The pathophysiology of fragile X syndrome involves inactivation of the *FMR-1* gene at Xq27.3, caused by multiple abnormal CGG base repeats.

What is the core feature of oppositional-defiant disorder?

Disrespectful to authority figures.

Short tempered, easy to become angry, resentful.

What is the first physical change during female sexual development?

A growth spurt in height.

What is the first step in evaluating a 2-year-old child who does not speak?

Check audiometry.

What is the main clinical presentation of pediatric autoimmune neuropsychiatric disorders associated with streptococcal infection (PANDAS)?

Choreiform movements.

Obsessive-compulsive symptoms.

What is the most common emergency diagnosis in child and adolescent psychiatry?

Threat of suicide.

What is the most effective treatment for conduct disorder?

Behavior therapy.

An effective behavior therapy plan for conduct disorder should include environmental structure and parent management training.

What is the most important domain in finding abnormalities for a diagnosis of autistic disorder?

Interpersonal relations and social interaction.

What is the most important prognostic factor related to long-term outcome in infantile autism?

Language development.

What medical conditions should be ruled out before making a diagnosis of encopresis?

Hirschsprung disease and other conditions that may cause fecal retention.

Physical examination, abdominal radiography, and fecal examination may be indicated.

What persons are legally required to report child abuse?

Teachers, physicians, district attorneys, and hospital activity therapists.

When young children need to be examined in the emergency room setting, should their parents be allowed to stay with them?

Yes, the presence of parents is usually appropriate.

This may also minimize the psychological trauma to the patient.

What are the characteristics of Asperger disorder, and how is it differentiated from autistic disorder or Kanner autism?

Asperger disorder is a disorder within the spectrum of autism. It is characterized by:

Poor social interaction (deficiencies in eye gaze, facial expression, body language, poor peer relationships, and lack of social reciprocity and interests).

A stereotyped or repetitive pattern of behavior.

Usually normal language development and intelligence quotient (IQ).

Autistic disorder, also known as Kanner autism, has the same symptoms as Asperger disorder, but is further marked by poor development in language and/or symbolic/imaginative play, and an IQ below 70 in 70% of cases.

CHAPTER 14 Psychosocial Therapies

What is "interpreting upward"?

A technique used to strengthen a patient's defenses and alleviate anxiety in supportive psychotherapy.

During psychotherapy, how does one tell the accuracy of a therapist's interpretation in regard to the patient's information?

The patient shows deepened insight when the therapist's interpretation is accurate.

According to object relations theory, what can conflict within a marriage generally be traced to?

Projective identification and splitting between the spouses.

How does the structural model of family therapy characterize the family?

A family is a complex system comprised of alliances and rivalries among family members.

After finishing the initial task of organizing planned meetings and selecting appropriate patients for supportive group therapy, what should the therapist do next?

Create and maintain a therapeutic environment, keeping in mind the culture of the group.

In psychotherapy, what could a psychiatrist's fear of experiencing the patient's rage and self-destructive behavior result in?

The psychiatrist becoming intimidated and helpless.

Give an example of "catastrophizing" in psychotherapy.	A patient who has an excellent working history fears being terminated in the next day's meeting with his supervisor.
What is overidentification?	The therapist feels great empathy toward the patient and fails to maintain sufficient distance to observe the patient's objective thoughts or behavior.
Give an example of confrontation.	"I think you'd rather talk about your job than face the sadness you felt in our last session."
What is the fundamental rule for psychoanalysis?	Free association.
What is working through?	A procedure in psychodynamic psychotherapy. Through the analyst's interpretation of transference and resistance, insight may finally become integrated into the patient's conscious awareness.
Besides being a conjunctive biologic treatment, does medication play a role in psychotherapy?	Medication prescribed by a psychiatrist may function as a psychological connection to the psychiatrist during the periods between visits.
What is the focus in interpersonal psychotherapy?	Patterns of communication.
For which patients is brief focal psychodynamic psychotherapy appropriate, and for which patients is it contraindicated?	Patients suitable for brief focal psychodynamic psychotherapy must be highly motivated, able to deal with psychological concepts, and able to develop a therapeutic alliance.

Contraindications to such therapy are past suicide attempts, substance dependence, chronic alcohol abuse, incapacitating obsessional or phobic symptoms, and destructive behavior.

Brief focal psychodynamic psychotherapy was developed at the Tavistock Clinic in London by Daniel Malan.

Why is group therapy often an appropriate therapy for adolescents?

Adolescents are more comfortable with peers, especially when they have to hear and consider critical comments. They also tend to dislike authority such as that of the therapist, which is diminished in group sessions.

What should a therapist do if a patient begins acting seductively and requests closer contact, such as an evening appointment or dinner?

The therapist should first examine his or her own behavior and possible counter-transference. Second, if appropriate, the therapist should discuss his or her observation with the patient and explore the meaning of the patient's behavior.

What conditions are considered appropriate for biofeedback therapy?

Neuromuscular conditions including pain, tension headaches, migraine headaches, neuromuscular rehabilitation, and seizure.

Cardiovascular conditions including hypertension, hypotension, cardiac arrhythmias, and Raynaud syndrome.

Gastrointestinal and genitourinary conditions including fecal incontinence and enuresis.

Pulmonary disease, consisting of asthma.

According to psychoanalytic theory, what is the etiology of the formation of a neurotic symptom?

Impaired ego function.

Failure of repression.

What factor correlates most strongly with a positive outcome of psychotherapy?

The therapist's empathy.

What is the essential technical goal of cognitive therapy?

Eliciting and testing automatic thoughts.

What is the therapeutic focus in supportive psychotherapy?

"Here and now"—coping with daily stresses.

What is double binding?

This concept, generated by Gregory Bateson, is used to describe a hypothetical family in which children receive conflicting parental messages about their behavior, attitudes, and feelings.

What are the five stages of reaction to approaching death developed by Elizabeth Kübler-Ross?

1. Shock and denial.
2. Anger.
3. Bargaining.
4. Depression.
5. Acceptance.

Treatment for a patient facing death is to recognize the reaction process and provide compassionate care.

What intervention techniques are utilized in a family-system approach to family therapy?

1. Giving the entire family specific homework assignments on which to work outside of treatment sessions.
2. Exploring the family's beliefs about the meaning of its members' behaviors.

3. Identifying family members' "problematic" behaviors and reframing them positively.
4. Directing members to engage in new behaviors during treatment sessions (e.g., changing seats), and observing the effects of this on patterns of behavior.

In the initial stage, the therapist should avoid identifying the most dysfunctional family dyad nor work on that relationship explicitly.

What is the primary focus of behavior therapy in the treatment of anorexia nervosa?

Restoring proper body weight.

What does the conceptual model of the "triangle of insight" involve?

Transference patterns, current relationships, and past relationships.

According to Daniel Malan, interpretation of the triangle of insight is the ideal goal in brief psychodynamic psychotherapy.

What should the psychiatrist do when 10 minutes late for an appointment with a psychodynamic psychotherapy patient?

Apologize and arrange to make up the time.

What is the most common theme discussed in psychotherapy with elderly patients?

Loss.

What is an example of countertransference?

A psychiatrist's not wanting to work with alcoholic patients, and believing that they are "hopeless" and "completely unmotivated."

When the meanings and effects of medications as well as their connecting function between therapist and the patient are integrated into the patient's understanding.

What type of psychotherapy should be more applicable to patients who have repeated "nervous breakdowns" under stress?

Supportive rather than insight-oriented psychotherapy.

What are the indications for a supportive emphasis in psychotherapy?

Poor frustration tolerance and severely impaired object relations.

What is confrontation?

It addresses an issue that the patient does not want to accept, or identifies the patient's avoidance or minimization of an issue. Although often gentle as practiced in psychotherapy, the concept of confrontation carries the unfortunate connotation in common parlance of aggressiveness or bluntness.

What is resistance?

Unconscious ideas or impulses that are repressed and prevented from reaching awareness because for some reason they are unacceptable to the patient's consciousness.

What are the indicators for termination in psychodynamic psychotherapy?

The superego has been modified, the presenting symptoms have been eliminated, the patient's interpersonal relationships have improved, and the patient is independently able to recognize and examine conflicts.

A separated couple is in marital therapy with a psychodynamically oriented therapist. How should the therapist demonstrate therapeutic neutrality in this case?

The concept of therapeutic neutrality is demonstrated by inquiring about why the couple is considering divorce, and also why they are considering returning to their marriage, if this is the case.

What is the indication for dialectical behavior therapy?

Borderline personality disorder.

Dialectical behavior therapy was developed by Marsha Linehan.

What is "reframing" in family therapy?

Also called "positive connotation," reframing is a relabeling of all negatively expressed feelings or behaviors as positive.

What psychotherapeutic technique is most important in the treatment of patients who are suicidal?

Establishing a therapeutic alliance.

CHAPTER 15 ECT, VNS, and DBS

What are the indications for electroconvulsive therapy (ECT)?

Well-established indications: Catatonia, major depressive disorder (MDD) (particularly psychotic depression), mania, acute psychosis. Medical intolerability to alternative treatment, patient request, and previous ECT responders are also considered first-line indications.

Possible indications: Delirium, obsessive-compulsive disorder (OCD), seizure, and Parkinson disease.

Not likely effective in: Somatization disorder, personality disorders, anxiety disorders (other than OCD), chronic status of schizophrenia.

Absolute contraindications: None.

Relative contraindications: Cardiovascular conditions, space-occupying intracranial lesions, cerebral aneurysms, recent strokes.

Which pattern of electrode placement for ECT is least likely to produce amnesia?

Unilateral at the nondominant side.

What conditions are indicated for treatment with vagus nerve stimulation (VNS)?

Medically refractory epilepsy.

Treatment-resistant depression.

How does one diagnose pseudocholinesterase deficiency?

Quick screening test: Acholest paper test.

Confirmation: Serum pseudocholinesterase activity.

Genotype: Allele-specific polymerase chain reaction, available only in advanced research laboratories.

Genetic consultation.

In deep brain stimulation (DBS), where are the usual locations electrodes are placed, and what are the major indications?

Thalamus for essential tremor and multiple sclerosis.

Globus pallidus or subthalamus for Parkinson disease.

What adverse effects may occur with the use of succinylcholine (Anectine) in ECT?

Muscle soreness due to fasciculation.

Increased extracellular potassium due to depolarization of the neuromuscular junction.

Prolonged apnea, particularly in patients with pseudocholinesterase deficiency.

What are the advantages of DBS compared to thalamotomy and pallidotomy?

Conservative and less destructive.

Easier surgery.

Safer and fewer side effects.

Adjustable dosage.

Preserves the potential for future treatment with more advanced techniques, such as brain cell transplantation.

What are the mechanisms of action of ECT?

Unknown.

The assumed primary therapeutic component is the bilateral spread of convulsion.

What are the risks of DBS?

Paralysis.

Changes in thinking, memory, and personality.

Seizures.

Infection.

What are the side effects of ECT?

Headache.

Confusion. Up to 10% of patients experience confusion within 30 minutes after treatment. The confusion usually resolves spontaneously.

Delirium. This typically clears within days.

Memory impairment. Almost all patients recover to baseline memory status after 6 months.

Cardiac arrhythmias. Usually mild and transient, it occurs more commonly in patients with cardiac disease. Usually induced by postictal vagal hyperactivity that causes bradycardia.

High blood pressure. Blood pressure increases transiently during seizures.

There is no evidence of ECT causing permanent brain damage.

What is ECT's effect on memory?

ECT is associated with both anterograde and retrograde amnesia.

More severe with bilateral ECT.

Usually brief; however, persistent memory difficulty for up to 6 months was reported.

What is the mortality rate of ECT?

Estimated at 0.01% to 0.03% per patient.

What is required or recommended for pre-ECT evaluation?

Medical and psychiatric history.

Physical examination.

Complete blood cell count.

Electrolytes.

Electrocardiogram.

Chest x-ray.

Other tests that are indicated for the patient's underlying medical condition.

What is the anesthetic agent of choice for ECT?

An agent with rapid onset and brief duration of action is most suitable.

Methohexital (Brevital) has been long accepted as the agent of choice by most ECT teams. *However, recently its limited availability has become a barrier to routine use.*

Propofol (Diprivan), etomidate (Amidate), and other alternative agents have been used.

What is the psychodynamic explanation of ECT's effect?

Psychodynamic schools once believed ECT may fulfill the need for punishment in depressed patients. This is, however, not substantiated by evidence.

What management is suitable if a patient with pseudocholinesterase deficiency was administered succinylcholine?

Mechanical ventilation is the first-line treatment. The longest reported paralytic effect is about 8 hours.

Genetic consultation and a medical alert bracelet may be considered.

What muscle relaxants are used in ECT?

Succinylcholine is the agent of choice due to its ease of use and low cost.

Atracurium (Tracrium) and mivacurium may be used alternatively in patients intolerant to succinylcholine (e.g., pseudocholinesterase deficiency) or with previous good experience with atracurium.

What neurophysiologic changes occur during the process of ECT?

Upregulation of norepinephrine and serotonin receptors.

Increase of the extracellular serotonin and norepinephrine concentration.

Rise in seizure threshold.

Increase in level of brain derived neurotrophic factor.

Possible increase in mossy fiber sprouting and neurogenesis in the hippocampus.

What side effects are common for VNS?

Hoarseness.

Coughing.

Paresthesia: Tingling or pain in the neck.

Dysphagia.

Dyspnea.

These side effects generally are mild and tend to go away over time.

What are the risks of VNS?

Injury to the vagus nerve.

Injury to the carotid artery and jugular vein.

Infection.

Bleeding.

Why is lithium recommended to be withheld during the course of ECT?

Lithium has been reported to be associated with severe prolonged postictal delirium.

Why is thalamic DBS not recommended for Parkinson disease?

Stimulation of the thalamus is effective only for tremor and rigidity, not the full spectrum of parkinsonian symptoms.

Stimulation of the globus pallidus and subthalamus provide improvement in the full range of Parkinson disease symptoms, including tremor, rigidity, slowness of movement, stiffness, and walking concerns. Therefore DBS on these two locations are recommended for Parkinson disease.

CHAPTER 16 Psychopharmacology

Which antidepressants cause no sexual dysfunction?

Bupropion, mirtazapine, and nefazodone. Duloxetine, a newer antidepressant, may have minimal sexual side effects as well.

What medication could psychiatrists use to treat patients with male sexual exhibitionism?

The first-line medication is medroxyprogesterone acetate.

Other medications including antidepressants and antipsychotics could also be used.

What receptor is related to mirtazapine's sedation and weight gain side effects?

Histamine 1 receptor.

What is the important pregnancy-related factor that influences a patient's lithium level?

Massive fluid shifts at the time of delivery.

Which atypical antipsychotic is unique by its inhibition of norepinephrine reuptake?

Ziprasidone.

Which atypical antipsychotics is a partial D2-receptor agonist?

Aripiprazole.

Which part of the brain is primarily involved in the synthesis of serotonin?

Raphe nuclei.

The cardiac effects of lithium most closely resemble which phenomenon on an electrocardiogram?

Hypokalemia.

What medication could significantly increase serum levels of paroxetine?

Cimetidine. It blocks the liver cytochrome P450 (CYP450) enzyme that metabolizes paroxetine.

What medication could significantly decrease the serum level of the medicine itself?

Carbamazepine. It induces the liver enzyme via an autoinduction mechanism to metabolize more medication.

What is the safety of antidepressants in pregnancy?

Because of the lack of convincing prospective data, this is not a fair question. Of note is that class B antidepressants have been found safe in animal studies, class C drugs have shown adverse effects in animal studies, and neither has established human safety. Because the vast majority of human studies have focused on SSRIs and tricyclic antidepressants (TCAs), these drugs are at least well tested. Therefore, SSRIs can be suggested for use during pregnancy, given their better side-effect profile (in pregnant women), with the exception of paroxetine.

Class B antidepressant maprotiline is the only one.

Class C antidepressants are SSRIs except paroxetine, MAOIs, bupropion, mirtazapine, and venlafaxine and all TCAs except those in class D named below.

Class D: Amitriptyline, imipramine, nortriptyline, and paroxetine.

Which antidepressants have adverse cardiac effects?

TCAs and trazodone.

Which antidepressants have strong sedative effects?

Amitriptyline, clomipramine, imipramine, mirtazapine, nefazodone, and trazodone.

Which antidepressants have weak or no anticholinergic effects?

SSRIs, bupropion, mirtazapine, nefazodone, trazodone, and venlafaxine. (TCAs and MAOIs have strong anticholinergic effects.)

What is the most frequent side effect of MAOIs?

Hypotension.

What is the treatment of choice for atypical depression?

MAOIs (phenelzine, tranylcypromine).

What are the contraindications to bupropion?

Seizure, eating disorders, and use of an MAOI within the previous 14 days.

Facts about MAOIs:

The most common side effect of MAOIs is orthostatic hypotension.

Foods that contain a high level of tyramine (e.g., red wine, aged cheese, nuts, chocolate) are contraindicated during the use of MAOIs.

MAOIs are contraindicated with the use of:

1. All other antidepressants. A 14-day (28-day for fluoxetine) systemic clearance period is necessary.
2. Meperidine.
3. Adrenergic agonists (e.g., phenylephrine, phenylpropanolamine).

Adrenergic antagonists such as phentolamine are not contraindicated with MAOIs.

Lithium is not contraindicated with MAOIs.

What is the clinical presentation of an MAOI-induced hypertensive crisis?

High blood pressure (BP), headache, stiff neck, and vomiting.

How should an MAOI-induced hypertensive crisis (BP = 240/140 mm Hg with a pounding headache) be treated?

1. The first-line treatment agent is an α-adrenergic blocking agent given intravenously (IV). Phentolamine (up to 5 mg IV) has been used.
2. Chlorpromazine (25 to 50 mg intramuscularly [IM] or orally [PO]) can be given as a second-line agent and is usually available.
3. Oral nifedipine can be given if there is early onset of a severe, bilateral, pounding occipital headache.

What is the pharmacologic mechanism of action of mirtazapine?

Central α2-adrenergic receptor antagonism. Since activation of α2-receptors inhibits the release of serotonin, mirtazapine can increase central serotonergic tone. In addition, mirtazapine blocks 5-hydroxytryptamine (serotonin) types

2 and 3 (5-HT_2 and 5-HT_3) receptors, and therefore increases the relative activity of 5-HT_{1a} and 5-HT_{1c} receptors.

The sedative effect of mirtazapine is caused by its antagonistic effect at the histamine 1 (H1) receptor. The sedative effect appears at a low dose, but may weaken at a higher dose.

What are the side effects and drug interactions of nefazodone?

1. Has no anticholinergic effects. (The only antidepressants that have moderate to severe anticholinergic effects are TCAs and MAOIs.)
2. Does not cause sexual dysfunction.
3. Is highly sedative.
4. Is a strong inhibitor of CYP450 3A4. Only triazolam is officially contraindicated for concurrent use with nefazodone.

Benzodiazepines metabolized by CYP450 3A4 and therefore not recommended for concurrent use with nefazodone are: M*idazolam,* a*lprazolam, and* t*riazolam (MAT). Diazepam is metabolized by both CYP450 3A4 and CYP450 2C19.*

What are the characteristics of serotonin syndrome?

It is caused by SSRIs or MAOIs, especially when these are combined with tyramine-containing foods.

The combination of MAOIs with meperidine is contraindicated. A 14-day washout period should be allowed when switching from MAOIs to other antidepressants.

Features of the serotonin syndrome are:

- Jitteriness, myoclonus, tremor at rest, hypertonicity, and rigidity.
- Autonomic instability (diaphoresis, hypo-/hypertension).
- Insomnia, excitement, coma, death.

What are the half-lives of various SSRIs?

Longest: Fluoxetine (7 to 15 days).

Shortest: Fluvoxamine (15 hours).

All other SSRIs: 1 day.

Fluoxetine is the only SSRI with clinically active metabolites (norfluoxetine).

What drug interactions occur with TCAs?

TCAs are metabolized by CYP450 2D6, 1A2, and 3A4.

Cigarette smoking, which induces CYP450 1A2, may decrease TCA concentrations.

Some antipsychotic agents (e.g., clozapine, haloperidol, risperidone, thioridazine) are competitors with TCAs for CYP450 2D6, and therefore increase TCA concentrations.

Methylphenidate decreases the metabolism of TCAs and therefore increases their concentrations.

Drugs that increase TCA levels are antipsychotics and methylphenidate.

Cigarette smoking decreases TCA levels.

What severe reactions have occurred with TCAs?

Cases of sudden death have been reported in children in association with the use of desipramine.

Overdosage with TCAs is associated with arrhythmia, seizure, delirium, and respiratory depression.

What is the best monitoring method to use for a patient who has overdosed on an unknown amount of a TCA?

Electrocardiography.

TCAs can potentially cause cardiac arrhythmia and death.

Which TCA has blood levels that are related to its clinical effect and needs to be monitored?

Nortriptyline.

The clinical therapeutic blood level for nortriptyline is 50 to 150 ng/mL.

What are the major effects and properties of venlafaxine?

Venlafaxine blocks reuptake of three neurotransmitters: Serotonin, norepinephrine, and dopamine.

It may cause increased diastolic BP.

Its half-life is very short among antidepressants (5 hours, and the half-life of its metabolite, desmethylvenlafaxine, 12 hours).

Venlafaxine does not inhibit CYP450.

What are the half-lives of various benzodiazepines?

Short (hours): Triazolam (Halcion), oxazepam (Serax). Benzodiazepines with short half-lives are associated with rebound insomnia when their use is discontinued.

Intermediate (<1 day): Alprazolam (Xanax), lorazepam (Ativan).

Long (>1 day): Clonazepam (Klonopin).

Very long (days): Diazepam (Valium), chlordiazepoxide (Librium).

What benzodiazepines are safe to use in patients with compromised hepatic function?

Temazepam, oxazepam, and lorazepam. These drugs do not need oxidation, and have no active metabolites.

TOL (*t*emazepam, *o*xazepam, and *l*orazepam).

What is the mechanism of action of benzodiazepines?

Benzodiazepines bind to binding sites (also known as benzodiazepine receptors) on receptors for γ-aminobutyric acid (GABA) and enhance the effects of GABA.

Benzodiazepine receptors are not independent receptors. They are specific binding sites located on GABA receptors.

Which benzodiazepines are available in parenteral form?

Four benzodiazepines have parenteral forms:

1. Chlordiazepoxide: Has multiple active metabolites (including diazepam), a medium rate of absorption, and a long duration of action.
2. Diazepam: Has multiple active metabolites, a rapid rate of absorption, and a long duration of action.
3. Lorazepam: Has no active metabolites, a reliably rapid-to-medium rate of absorption, and a short duration of action.
4. Midazolam: This drug is available for IV injection, has active metabolites, and has a short duration of action.

What is the drug of first choice in the treatment of catatonia?

A benzodiazepine. The most commonly used agent is lorazepam given IM.

What are the major differences in side-effect profiles of typical low-potency and typical high-potency antipsychotic agents?

Low-potency agents are more likely to cause hypotension, anticholinergic effects, and sedation, and less likely to cause extrapyramidal side effects (EPS).

High-potency agents are more likely to cause EPS and less likely to cause hypotension, anticholinergic effects, and sedation.

Commonly used typical antipsychotic agents:

High potency: Haloperidol (Haldol), fluphenazine (Prolixin).

Medium potency: Molindone (Moban), loxapine (Loxitane).

Low potency: Chlorpromazine (Thorazine), thiothixene (Navane).

Elderly persons are more sensitive to anticholinergic effects, and may become confused when given an antipsychotic agent.

What are the treatment modalities for neuroleptic malignant syndrome (NMS)?

Discontinue antipsychotics, hydration (IV fluids), cooling, dantrolene, and bromocriptine (Parlodel).

What are anticholinergic effects?

Symptoms: Dryness of the mouth, urinary retention, decreased bronchial secretion, tachycardia, and constipation. Memory impairment may occur at toxic doses.

Treatment: Bethanechol (Urecholine), or reduce anticholinergic drug dosage.

Psychiatric medicines with anticholinergic effects are:

1. Among antipsychotic agents, clozapine (Clozaril), thioridazine, and mesoridazine (Serentil) have strong anticholinergic effects. All other antipsychotic agents have weak cholinergic effects.
2. Among antidepressants, TCAs and MAOIs have strong anticholinergic effects. All other antidepressants have weak anticholinergic effects.

Other drugs that have anticholinergic effects include antiparkinsonian agents such as benztropine (Cogentin).

What is the side-effect profile of clozapine?

The most common side effect is sedation.

Important severe reactions are seizures, agranulocytosis, and NMS.

Other common side effects are hypotension, headache, hyperglycemia, and weight gain.

Clozapine has a minimal effect on prolactin level.

What are the clinical features of NMS?

General: Altered consciousness, fever, and mutism.

Autonomic: Labile blood pressure, tachycardia, diaphoresis, incontinence, dysphasia.

Muscular: Rigidity, tremor.

Hematologic: Leukocytosis, elevated creatine kinase.

What is the mechanism by which NMS occurs?

Blockade of dopamine receptors in the basal ganglia, hypothalamus, postganglionic sympathetic neurons, and smooth muscle. NMS may also involve blockade of nondopamine monoamines.

Besides being caused by typical antipsychotic agents, NMS may also be caused by TCA, SSRI, and atypical antipsychotic agents.

The risk of NMS is increased with use of lithium and sudden discontinuation of levodopa.

What are the important drug interactions of carbamazepine?

Carbamazepine induces liver enzymes that increase its own metabolism and may also reduce the effectiveness of other medicines such as oral contraceptives. As a result of this effect, the serum level of carbamazepine may drop over a period of months. Periodic reassessment of the carbamazepine serum level is therefore necessary, and its dosage should be adjusted accordingly.

The concentration of carbamazepine is increased with concurrent use of cimetidine.

Liver-enzyme induction: Carbamazepine.

Liver-enzyme inhibition: Cimetidine.

What are the important drug interactions of lithium?

Drugs that increase lithium levels are angiotensin-converting enzyme inhibitors, fluoxetine, ibuprofen (Motrin), indomethacin (Indocin), and diuretics (spironolactone, thiazide).

Drugs that decrease lithium levels are theophylline, caffeine, and laxatives.

What are the effects of lithium intoxication?

Cardiac: ST-segment depression and QT-interval prolongation on the electrocardiogram.

Neuromuscular: Ataxia, coarse tremor, dysarthria, and epilepsy.

Kidney: Nephrotoxicity (interstitial fibrosis).

Thyroid: None. Lithium may cause hypothyroidism. This is a side effect that remits when lithium is discontinued. Lithium is not thyrotoxic.

Treatment: Supportive; hemodialysis if the serum lithium level is above 4.0 mmol/L.

What are the mechanisms of action of lithium?

1. Lithium does not work at the synapse through effects of neurotransmitters.
2. Lithium works at the level of G-proteins and other second messengers, such as phosphatidylinositol phosphate (PIP).

Current hypotheses: Lithium blocks the G-protein–mediated transmission of messages through:

1. Inhibition of inositol monophosphate phosphatase (IMPase).

2. Inhibition of the α unit of G-proteins.
3. Inhibition of glycogen synthase kinase-3β (GSK-3β).
4. Inhibition of adenylyl cyclase.

How is lithium metabolized?

Lithium is not metabolized, and its half-life does not change with impaired hepatic function. Lithium is excreted via the kidney.

What are the side effects of lithium?

1. Tremor: This may occur at therapeutic levels of lithium.

Treatment involves dividing the dose, reducing coffee intake, or use of a β-blocker (propranolol).

2. Polyuria/polydipsia (nephrogenic diabetes insipidus [DI]): Is treated with amiloride, a potassium-sparing diuretic that inhibits sodium resorption at the distal convoluted tubule.
3. Weight gain: Caused by increased caloric intake.
4. Hypothyroidism: Lithium inhibits iodine uptake, iodination of tyrosine, and the release of triiodothyronine (T_3) and thyroxine (T_4).
5. Rash.

Lithium has no adverse effects on the respiratory system.

What factors are important in maintenance treatment with lithium?

A dramatic change in the sodium serum concentration may change the serum lithium concentration. It is important to maintain usual sodium and fluid intake during lithium treatment.

Massive fluid shifts (pregnancy/labor) may change lithium concentrations.

Close monitoring of lithium levels is required in patients with unstable renal function or congestive heart disease.

Which psychiatric medicine may cause nephrogenic DI?

Lithium. DI is not associated with other psychiatric medicines.

Please note that the syndrome of inappropriate secretion of antidiuretic hormone (SIADH) is associated with many psychiatric medicines.

DI: Lack of antidiuretic hormone (ADH), also known as vasopressin, or a poor renal response to ADH. SIADH is marked by an abnormally high level of ADH.

ADH acts at the renal collecting tubules to enhance free-water resorption.

Which thyroid function test should be repeated at 6 months for patients taking lithium?

Thyroid-stimulating hormone (TSH).

What is the treatment of choice for rapidly cycling mood disorder?

Anticonvulsant agents, such as valproic acid.

What are the side effects of valproic acid?

Common: Weight gain, hair loss.

Less common: Thrombocytopenia, bone-marrow suppression.

Congenital defects: Neural tube, cardiac, limb, and facial, and hypospadias.

Hirsutism: Phenytoin.

Hair loss: Valproic acid.

What laboratory test is needed in carbamazepine-treated patients at 2-week intervals during the first 2 months of treatment?

A complete blood cell count (CBC) for the early detection of blood dyscrasias, such as aplastic anemia, agranulocytosis, leukopenia, and thrombocytopenia.

Also, liver function tests to detect drug-induced hepatitis.

What medicines have inhibitory effects on CYP450 enzymes?

Nefazodone, fluvoxamine, and TCAs: High inhibition of CYP450 3A4.

Sertraline, fluoxetine: Low inhibition of CYP450 3A4.

Paroxetine, fluoxetine: High inhibition of CYP450 2D6.

TCAs, sertraline: Low inhibition of CYP450 2D6.

Benzodiazepines metabolized by CYP450 3A4 are midazolam, alprazolam, and triazolam.

Diazepam is metabolized by both CYP450 3A4 and CYP450 2C19.

Triazolam is contraindicated for concurrent use with nefazodone.

Which drugs cause drug-induced delayed ejaculation and retrograde ejaculation?

Drugs with α-adrenergic antagonistic effects. Most typical antipsychotics have significant antagonistic effects on α-adrenergic receptors. Drugs known to have such side effects include thioridazine and chlorpromazine.

What are the causes of EPS, and how are they treated?

Mechanisms: EPS are theoretically attributed to blockade of dopamine-2 (D2) receptors in the nigrostriatal pathway, and to these receptors' subsequent supersensitivity.

Treatment:

Akathisia: Propranolol.

Acute dystonia: Benztropine or diphenhydramine (Benadryl).

What are the core features of neuroleptic-induced dystonia?

Abnormal positioning or spasm of the muscles of the head, neck, limbs, or trunk, developing within a few days of starting a neuroleptic medication or raising its dose.

Neuroleptic-induced parkinsonism is marked by a parkinsonian tremor, muscular rigidity, or akinesia developing within a few weeks of starting a neuroleptic medication or raising its dose.

Neuroleptic-induced akathisia is marked by subjective complaints of restlessness accompanied by observed movements (e.g., fidgety movements of the legs, rocking from foot to foot, pacing, or inability to sit or stand still) developing within a few weeks of starting a neuroleptic medication or raising its dose.

Neuroleptic-induced tardive dyskinesia is marked by involuntary choreiform, athetoid, or rhythmic movements (lasting at least a few weeks) of the tongue, jaw, or extremities, and developing in association with the use of neuroleptic medication for at least a few months.

What is meperidine?	An analgesic agent. Meperidine may cause seizure, and is contraindicated with use of MAOIs.
What are the symptoms of benztropine intoxication?	Crazy: Agitation, hallucinations. Dry: Dry skin, dry mouth. Red: Flushing, hyperthermia. Hypotension, tachycardia, mydriasis (dilated pupils), decreased bowel sounds, seizure, delirium, and coma.
Which typical antipsychotic agent is least likely to cause weight gain?	Molindone.
What is the mechanism of orthostatic hypotension?	Blockade of α_1-adrenergic receptors.
What psychiatric medications cause priapism?	Priapism is a rare but important side effect of trazodone. Other medicines that may cause priapism include venlafaxine, levodopa, and sildenafil.
Retinal pigmentation is an adverse effect of which antipsychotic agent?	Retinal pigmentation may be associated with the use of thioridazine (Mellaril) at high doses (above 800 mg/d).
What are some risk factors for tardive dyskinesia?	Old age, mood disorder, female gender, childhood, African American heritage, and diabetes.

What are some indications for psychostimulants?

Attention-deficit/hyperactivity disorder (ADHD).

Narcolepsy.

Exogenous obesity.

Depression in elderly and medically ill persons.

Psychostimulants should not be used in personality disorders or for patients with a history of substance abuse.

What are the choices of pharmacologic treatment for ADHD?

Stimulants: Methylphenidate (Ritalin) is usually the drug of first choice. Dextroamphetamine (Dexedrine) and amphetamine (Adderall) may be used as drugs of first choice or alternatives. Pemoline (Cylert) may cause liver failure.

Antidepressants: Bupropion (Wellbutrin) and other antidepressants.

Clonidine.

How are β-blockers used in psychiatry?

β-blockers have been less frequently used in psychiatric treatment in recent years than formerly. They are still useful in the treatment of social phobia. They are also used to reduce or reverse side effects caused by other psychopharmacologic treatment, such as lithium-induced postural tremor and neuroleptic-induced acute akathisia.

What drug interactions occur with cimetidine?

Cimetidine inhibits liver enzymes, and increases the serum concentration of many drugs, including:

SSRIs.

Benzodiazepines.

Anticonvulsants (carbamazepine, phenytoin, valproic acid derivatives).

β-blockers.

TCAs.

Sildenafil (Viagra).

What is the first-pass effect?

Initial metabolism of a drug within the portal circulation of the liver before the drug reaches the systemic circulation.

What are some metabolic characteristics of geriatric patients?

Increased fat.

Decreased hepatic metabolism, intestinal motility, plasma-binding proteins (albumin), glomerular filtration rate, and renal clearance.

What pharmacologic treatment is available for obsessive-compulsive disorder (OCD)?

Antidepressants with serotonergic effects, such as SSRIs, clomipramine, and MAOIs. High doses are needed. Antidepressants without serotonergic effects, such as bupropion, are not effective.

How is seasonal depression diagnosed and treated?

Seasonal depression is diagnosed with the *Diagnostic and Statistical Manual of Mental Disorders, Fourth Edition*, by applying a seasonal pattern specifier to major depressive disorder (MDD) or bipolar disorders.

The treatment for seasonal depression is phototherapy.

What are the indications for electroconvulsive therapy (ECT)?

Well-established indications for ECT are: Catatonia, MDD, mania, and schizophrenia (acute psychosis).

Other indications: Delirium, OCD, seizure, and Parkinson disease.

ECT is not effective in: somatization disorder, personality disorders, anxiety disorders.

ECT is usually not effective in: Chronic schizophrenia.

Absolute contraindications: None.

Relative contraindications: Cardiovascular conditions, space-occupying intracerebral lesions, cerebral aneurysms, recent strokes.

What are the mechanisms of action of ECT?

They are unknown. The assumed primary therapeutic component is the bilateral spread of convulsion.

What medicines should be discontinued before ECT is given?

Lithium and benzodiazepines.

What are the side effects of ECT?

1. Headache.
2. Confusion: Up to 10% of patients experience confusion within 30 minutes after treatment; this usually resolves spontaneously.
3. Delirium: This typically clears within days.
4. Memory impairment: No permanent brain damage. Almost all patients recover to baseline memory status after 6 months.

5. Cardiac arrhythmias: Mild and transient, occurring more commonly in patients with cardiac disease. Usually induced by post-ictal vagal hyperactivity that causes bradycardia.
6. High blood pressure: Blood pressure increases transiently during seizures.

Which psychiatric drugs require routine monitoring of their serum levels?

Lithium, desipramine, nortriptyline, valproic acid, and carbamazepine.

What medications are effective for the treatment of panic disorder?

Benzodiazepines.

TCAs.

MAOIs.

SSRIs and SNRIs.

What was the first psychiatric medicine to be introduced into clinical use?

Chlorpromazine, introduced in 1953.

Other landmark agents in psychopharmacology:

First mood stabilizer: Lithium, introduced in 1949.

First antidepressant: TCAs, particularly tofranil, introduced in 1957.

First SSRI: Fluoxetine (Prozac), introduced in 1985.

Withdrawal from what substance may cause grand mal seizure as well as severe anxiety and insomnia?

Alcohol.

Benzodiazepines.

Barbiturates.

Meprobamate.

Meprobamate is a nonbenzodiazepine anxiolytic agent with muscle-relaxant properties.

What pharmacologic agents are usually used to manage acute violent episodes in the emergency department setting?

Haloperidol and benzodiazepine.

New medications include ziprasidone and olanzapine IM.

PART III

CLINICAL NEUROLOGY

CHAPTER 17 Seizure Disorders

What clinical feature can differentiate complex partial seizures from simple partial seizures?

Complex partial seizures are marked by an altered responsiveness to outside stimuli without loss of consciousness.

In simple partial seizures there is no change in responsiveness to outside stimuli.

For pregnant women with epilepsy, what important issues should be discussed?

Increased rate of polycystic ovarian syndrome.

Reduced fertility rate.

Seizures during pregnancy may cause hypoxia to the fetus.

Teratogenic antiepileptics: Carbamazepine, valproate, phenytoin.

Is the direction of eye deviation during a seizure related to the location of the seizure focus?

Yes. During a seizure, the eyes deviate in the direction of the seizure focus.

Post-ictally, the eyes deviate away from the seizure focus.

The principle is, the eyes always look in the direction of the excited neuron.

What antiepileptic drugs induce hepatic metabolism and therefore reduce efficacy of oral contraceptives?

Barbiturates (Luminal).

Carbamazepine (Tegretal, Carbatrol).

Lamotrigine.

Oxcarbazepine (Trileptal).

Phenytoin (Dilantin).

Topiramate (Topamax).

What antiepileptics can cause liver impairment?

Carbamazepine.

Valproate (Depakote, Depakene, Depacon).

What are clinical features of absence epilepsy?

It is considered a generalized seizure because of loss of consciousness. Almost always occurs in children.

Abrupt loss and quick resolution of consciousness, no post-ictal state. Automatisms such as blinking, lip smacking.

Average duration <10 seconds.

May be induced by hyperventilation.

Pathognomonic electroencephalogram (EEG): 3-Hz spike and wave.

What are concerns in prescribing antiepileptics in women of childbearing age?

Polycystic ovarian syndrome (valproate).

Hyperandrogenism (valproate).

Reducing effectiveness of oral contraceptives (phenytoin and carbamazepine).

Fetal neural tube defects (valproate).

Which anticonvulsants do not have hepatic metabolism?

Gabapentin (Neurontin).

Levetiracetam (Keppra).

Topiramate has minimal hepatic metabolism.

What are features of partial and focal seizures with regard to anatomic location of brain pathology?

Primary motor cortex: Contralateral motor tonic-clonic seizures.

Supplementary motor cortex: Complex bizarre automatisms (facial muscle seizures often mistaken for psychosis).

Occipital lobe: Elementary visual hallucinations, ictal amaurosis (blindness).

Parietal lobe: Contralateral paresthesias, pain, gustatory hallucinations, language disturbances if seizure is from dominant lobe.

Mesial temporal lobe: Abdominal complaints, often an aura of focal seizures.

Superior temporal lobe: Auditory hallucinations, often an aura of focal seizures.

What is the first-line treatment for partial seizures?

Carbamazepine.

What are the clinical features of complex partial epilepsy of temporal lobe origin?

Consciousness is impaired but not lost.

Epigastric sensations are most common, but affective (fear), cognitive (déjà vu), and sensory (olfactory hallucinations) may occur.

Seizures generally last for less than 30 minutes, average 1 to 3 minutes.

The motor manifestation of complex partial epilepsy is termed "automatism," which takes the form of orobuccolingual movements in about 75% of patients, and other facial or neck movements in about 50%.

What are possible complications of epilepsy surgery?

Bleeding.

Infection.

Functional deficit.

What are the side effects of phenytoin?

Dose-related side effects:

Diplopia, ataxia, gingival hyperplasia, hirsutism (in contrast to another antiepileptic, valproic acid, which may cause hair loss), coarse facial features, polyneuropathy, osteomalacia, and megaloblastic anemia.

Idiosyncratic side effects:

Skin rash, fever, lymphoid hyperplasia, hepatic dysfunction, blood dyscrasia, and Stevens-Johnson syndrome.

What is the first-line medication for childhood absence epilepsy?

Ethosuximide (Zarontin).

What features of pseudoseizure are helpful in distinguishing it from genuine seizure?

No tonic phase (synchronous limb thrashing).

No real loss of consciousness or behavioral automatism, though there may be apparent "loss of consciousness."

No post-ictal confusion.

No urinary incontinence.

No seizure activity in EEG.

No elevation of serum prolactin level. Serum prolactin level elevates in 1 hour after a generalized tonic-clonic or partial complex seizure.

What is Jacksonian seizure?

A simple partial seizure that may spread to contiguous regions of the motor cortex.

Also known as "Jacksonian march."

What physical signs should raise the concern of antiepileptic intoxication?

Ataxia of gait.

Dysarthria.

Dysmetria on heel-shin testing.

Lethargy.

Nystagmus.

Tremor.

Which anticonvulsants can cause renal stones?

Topiramate.

Zonisamide (Zonegran).

What psychotropic medicines increase risk of seizures?

Amoxapine.

Bupropion (Wellbutrin).

Chlorpromazine (Thorazine).

Clozapine (Clozaril): <300 mg/d 1%, >600 mg/d 4.4%.

Loxapine (Loxitane).

What psychiatric conditions may present as comorbidities in patients with epilepsy?

Depression: Presents in 20% to 50% of seizure patients, and is highest in left temporal complex partial epilepsy. Risk factors include late onset of seizures, left temporal hypometabolism, and right hemisphere epilepsy surgery.

Anxiety: Presents in 20% to 60% of patients, and is highest in intractable epilepsy. Focal seizures may present as panic attacks.

Psychosis: Inter-ictal and post-ictal psychosis. Risk factors are family history of psychosis, younger age of onset, low IQ, bilateral independent foci, and mood disorders among first-degree relatives.

Suicide: Annual suicidal rate among epileptic patients is five times that of the general population, with temporal lobe epilepsy having the highest rate—twenty-five times! Ictal command hallucination is a major risk factor.

What seizure conditions may be improved by epilepsy surgery?

Focal cortical dysplasia.

Hemimegalencephaly.

Isolated structural lesions: Dysembryoplastic tumors, low-grade astrocytomas, vascular abnormalities.

Mesial temporal sclerosis.

Tuberous sclerosis.

Which anticonvulsants block both Na^+ and Ca^{2+} channels, and also enhance γ-aminobutyric acid activity?

Topiramate.

Gabapentin.

A 5-year-old child was observed to suddenly stop all activities for several seconds, and to blink his eyes. No confusion was found. What is the probable diagnosis?

Absence seizure, usually presents as brief loss of consciousness, no loss of postural tone, subtle motor manifestations (eye blinking, head turning), and rare automatisms. Also known as "petit mal seizure."

Usually begins in childhood, and does not persist after age 20 years.

May be induced by hyperventilation.

Recovers immediately with full orientation.

Treatment: Ethosuximide and valproic acid.

Which anticonvulsants can cause bone impairment?

Carbamazepine: Osteoporosis.

Phenobarbital: Osteomalacia.

Phenytoin: Osteomalacia.

Valproate: Osteomalacia.

Which anticonvulsants have a risk of causing bone marrow suppression?

Carbamazepine.

Ethosuximide.

Valproate.

Phenytoin.

Which anticonvulsants may cause change in body hair?

Valproate: Alopecia.

Phenytoin: Hirsutism.

Which anticonvulsants may cause Stevens-Johnson syndrome?

Phenytoin.

Carbamazepine.

Ethosuximide.

Lamotrigine.

Which antidepressant is structurally similar to carbamazepine?

Imipramine.

Due to this structural similarity, carbamazepine is sometimes prescribed in patients with both epilepsy and depression.

Which antiepileptic drug can cause polycystic ovarian syndrome?

Valproate.

Which antiepileptic drugs have a possible side effect of causing hyponatremia?

Carbamazepine.

Oxcarbazepine.

CHAPTER 18 Localized Impairment: Strokes, Brain Injuries, and Brain Tumors

What is the major ocular symptom of carotid insufficiency?

Transient monocular blindness.

What is anosognosia?

A body image disorder in which the patient neglects or fails to recognize part of his or her own body.

Usually takes the form of unilateral neglect.

Caused by a parietal lobe lesion.

The patient tends not to use the contralateral limbs, may deny that there is anything wrong with these limbs, and may even fail to recognize the contralateral limbs.

What are the clinical manifestations of an embolic stroke in the left angular gyrus?

Fluent speech and excellent comprehension.

Unable to name fingers and body parts nor to determine right or left orientation.

Unable to write down thoughts and take notes.

Good reading comprehension.

Unable to do calculations.

What language deficiency is typical in a stroke by occlusion of the anterior branches of the left middle cerebral artery?

Location is the inferior frontal convolution, including the Broca area.

Impaired fluency of spontaneous speech.

Which comorbid disease of AIDS produces cerebral focal lesions?

Toxoplasmosis.

Lymphoma.

What are the clinical features of myasthenia gravis?

Insidious onset. Slowly progressive course.

Diplopia, ptosis, dysarthria, extremity weakness, generalized weakness, dysphagia.

Weakness does not conform to the distribution of any single nerve.

Pupillary responses are not affected. Persistent activity of a muscle group leads to temporarily increased weakness, with restoration of strength after a brief rest.

What are the clinical findings in cases of upper motor neuron lesions?

Weakness, paralysis, spasticity.

Increased tendon reflexes, positive Babinski reflex.

No significant muscle atrophy.

What are the contraindications to the use of tissue plasminogen activator (tPA) for thrombolysis in acute stroke?

Risk of hemorrhage:

Prior intracranial hemorrhage; seizure at the onset of stroke symptoms; stroke or trauma occurring less than 3 months before the presenting stroke; a major surgical procedure within 14 days; gastrointestinal or urinary tract bleeding within 21 days; systolic blood pressure over 185 mm Hg or diastolic blood pressure over 110 mm Hg; current treatment with warfarin for atrial fibrillation.

To avoid unnecessary treatment:

Do not give tPA if neurologic deficits are improving rapidly and spontaneously; if deficits are mild and isolated; in the presence of hypo- or hyperglycemia (which can cause symptoms mimicking a stroke); when symptoms have begun more than 3 hours before the proposed tPA therapy.

Note: The patient's initial clinical symptoms (change in consciousness, headache, agitation, etc.) are usually not influential factors in the decision to undertake tPA treatment.

What are the lesion locations and clinical characteristics of aphasia?

Frontal lobe: Broca aphasia, also called expressive or nonfluent aphasia.

Good comprehension but poor repetition and fluency; paucity of speech; halting, agrammatic speech; telegraphic speech; may be associated with hemiparesis.

Posterior temporal lobe: Wernicke aphasia (receptive, fluent aphasia).

Good speech fluency but poor comprehension and poor repetition; intact grammar; neologisms; paraphasias; word salad; nonsensical speech; may be associated with a reduction in the visual field.

Arcuate fasciculus: Conduction aphasia.

Good speech comprehension and fluency; poor repetition.

What are the pathognomonic features of subarachnoid hemorrhage?

Sudden severe headache, relative preservation of consciousness, lack of focal signs, neck stiffness. Possible collapse.

What are the pros and cons of computed tomography (CT) and magnetic resonance imaging (MRI) of the head?

CT: Economical; more widely available; suitable for those with pacemakers; the diagnostic procedure of choice for acute hemorrhage or acute trauma.

MRI: Better differentiation of white from gray matter; better identification of white-matter lesions; better detection of posterior fossa and brainstem pathology; suitable for patients for whom radiation exposure is contraindicated (e.g., during pregnancy).

What brain tumors are common in adults but rare in children?

Glioblastoma multiforme.

Metastatic tumors.

What brain tumors are common in both children and adults?

Astrocytoma, which is relatively more common in children.

What cerebral areas are often involved in closed-head contusions with loss of consciousness?

The bases of the frontal lobes.

The tips of the temporal lobes.

What is "locked-in syndrome"?

A result of functional transection of the brainstem below the mid-pons.

Such patients are mute and quadriplegic, but do not lose consciousness, because the reticular formation lies above the level of the mid-pons.

Eye movement is intact.

Causes include infarct, hemorrhage, myelinolysis, tumor, and encephalitis.

What is internuclear ophthalmoplegia?

Internuclear ophthalmoplegia presents as disconjugate gaze with impaired adduction and nystagmus of the abducted eye.

When the patient attempts to look to the left, the left eye turns to the left with nystagmus, and the right eye cannot turn to the left. Vice versa when the patient attempts to look to the right.

The location of the lesion is the medial longitudinal fasciculus.

Most common causes:

In young adults: Multiple sclerosis.

In older patients: Vascular diseases.

What is the cerebral location for olfactory hallucinations followed by altered consciousness and orofacial automatisms?

Anterior medial temporal lobe.

How does one treat subacute combined degeneration?

Intramuscular vitamin B12.

What symptoms present in frontal lobe syndromes?

Orbitofrontal: Disinhibition and impulsiveness.

Medial frontal: Apathy.

Left frontal: Depression.

Right frontal: Mania.

What is Wallenberg syndrome?

Lateral medullary infarction. The clinical features vary, depending on the extent of infarction.

Structures affected and the corresponding clinical features are:

Vestibular nuclei: Vertigo, nystagmus.

Inferior cerebellar peduncle: Hemiataxia.

Spinal tract and nucleus of trigeminal nerve: Impairment of sensory modalities over the face.

Descending sympathetic tract: Ipsilateral Horner syndrome.

Spinothalamic tract: Loss of light and position sense in the ipsilateral limbs, impairment of pinprick and temperature sensation in the contralateral limbs.

Dorsal motor nucleus of the vagus nerve: Nausea, vomiting, dysphagia, and hoarseness.

What language deficiency is typical in a stroke in the inferior frontal convolution?

Impaired fluency of spontaneous speech (Broca aphasia);

Most likely caused by occlusion of the anterior branches of the left middle cerebral artery.

What treatments are available for acute strokes?

Ischemic strokes:

Thrombolysis: Must be done in 4 to 6 hours;

Heparin;

Physical therapy.

Hemorrhagic strokes:

Neurosurgery;

Conservative management: Close monitoring for continued bleeding and mass effect;

Vitamin K, avoid anticoagulants.

What types of hallucinations can be manifestations of central nervous system lesions?

Auditory hallucinations: Temporal lobe and pontine lesions;

Visual hallucinations: Occipital cortex lesions;

Peduncular hallucinosis: Also known as Lhermitte peduncular hallucinosis (named after French neurologist Jean Lhermitte).

A rare form of visual hallucination characterized by vivid visual images of people, animals, and plants, accompanied by sleep disturbances.

Associated with the upper brainstem and midbrain.

The clinical syndrome may include localizing signs. However, In the absence of localizing focal neurologic deficits, it is easily confused with a delirium or psychosis.

What visual impairment may present in the case of a lesion in the optic tract?

Contralateral homonymous hemianopsia.

The optic tract is connected to the ipsilateral retina, which reflects the contralateral visual field.

What visual lesion is likely to be caused by a pituitary tumor?

Bitemporal hemianopia.

When should anticoagulants be used in cerebrovascular diseases?

Indicated in:

TIA (transient ischemic attack) or completed stroke with a cardiac source.

Consider in:

Stroke in evolution;

TIA or completed stroke with a carotid or vertebrobasilar artery source.

CHAPTER 19 Peripheral Nerve and Muscle Disorders

What are the causes and symptoms of radial nerve injury?

Often due to prolonged compression of the arm. Typical causes are overdose and alcohol intoxication.

Motor paresis: Wrist drop—paresis of wrist and thumb extensors.

Sensory loss and pain: Dorsum of hand.

Loss of deep tendon reflex: Brachioradialis.

A patient develops progressive weakness 2 weeks after a viral infection. What is the possible diagnosis and what laboratory tests can be used to confirm it?

Guillain-Barré syndrome is also known as acute idiopathic inflammatory polyneuropathy.

Acute onset.

Symmetric weakness, usually beginning in the legs, and more marked proximally than distally.

Some sensory complaints.

Typical absence of deep tendon reflexes. There may be marked autonomic dysfunction.

Nerve conduction study: Slow conduction velocity, prolonged distal motor latency, and conduction blockade.

Cerebrospinal fluid (CSF): Increased protein concentration but a normal cell count.

How does botulinum toxin work in the treatment of blepharospasm, dystonic dysphonia, and torticollis?

It prevents the release of acetylcholine vesicles from presynaptic nerve terminals. In this way it reduces muscle spasm.

What are the electrophysiologic signs of muscle denervation?

Fibrillations.

Positive sharp waves.

What are the characteristics of carpal tunnel syndrome?

Pain and sensory deficits of the palmar surface.

Sensory deficits are confined to the median nerve distribution, and primarily involve the thumb, the index and middle fingers, and the lateral half of the ring finger.

Weakness in abduction of the thumb.

Pain in the arm.

Causes: Compression of the median nerve due to myxedema (from hypothyroidism), pregnancy, trauma, and other conditions.

What are the characteristics of ulnar nerve dysfunction?

The ulnar nerve is particularly susceptible to mechanical injury at the elbow by adjacent anatomic structures.

Also known as "ulnar nerve entrapment."

Clinical presentations include: Pain, sensory loss, and weakness, located in the fourth and fifth fingers and the ulnar border of the hand.

What are the common causes of carpal tunnel syndrome?

Myxedema (from hypothyroidism).

Pregnancy.

Repetitive stress injuries (typing, using a screwdriver, prolonged driving).

Trauma.

What is Guillain-Barré syndrome?

Named after two French neurologists, who among other things, contributed to the initial identification of the condition.

Acute inflammatory demyelinating polyradiculoneuropathy, also known as postinfectious demyelinating polyneuropathy.

Paresthesia and numbness starting in the fingers and toes, with quick involvement of the feet and legs, hands, arms, and respiratory muscles, and cranial nerves.

Symptoms often follow an upper respiratory or gastrointestinal (most often *Campylobacter jejuni*) illness. Could be idiopathic.

CSF: High protein and nearly normal cell counts.

Treatment is supportive.

What is the most effective treatment for focal dystonia?

Botulinum toxin.

What is the treatment for trigeminal neuralgia, also known as tic douloureux?

Carbamazepine can induce remission of symptoms in 24 hours.

Phenytoin will abort an acute attack.

What procedure should be chosen to diagnose spinal cord compression?

Magnetic resonance imaging.

What symptoms are typical for carpal tunnel syndrome?

Pain and sensory deficits (paresthesias).

Symptoms located at the palmar surface, and confined to the median nerve distribution (thumb, index and middle fingers, and the lateral half of the ring finger).

Weakness in abduction of the thumb.

Possible pain in the arm.

What treatment is appropriate for carpal tunnel syndrome?

Splints.

Diuretics.

Steroid injections.

Surgery to unroof the tunnel.

What treatments are available for Guillain-Barré syndrome?

Plasmapheresis.

Intravenous immunoglobulin.

Supportive therapy.

What is diabetic mononeuropathy simplex?

A condition likely to stem from the involvement of a cranial nerve.

The likelihood of involvement follows the order: Oculomotor (III), abducens (VI), and trochlear (IV).

The presentation involves a diabetic patient who has a periorbital headache of sudden onset on the right and diplopia of new onset.

Examination shows right eyelid ptosis and an inability to adduct or elevate the right eye. The pupils react normally to light directly and consensually. There is no pallor of the optic disk.

What are the clinical features of diabetic neuropathy?

Sensory deficits, including pain and paresthesia.

Motor deficits, presenting as muscle weakness and atrophy.

Autonomic neuropathy, presenting as postural hypotension, neurogenic bladder, and incontinence.

CHAPTER 20

Cranial Nerve Symptoms and Disorders

How does vertigo differ from syncope?

Vertigo is the illusion of movement of the body or the environment. It is caused by lesions affecting the labyrinth of the inner ear, the vestibular division of the auditory nerve, or brainstem vestibular nuclei.

Syncope results from the impaired brain supply of blood, oxygen, or glucose.

What are clinical features for benign positional vertigo?

Brief, severe vertigo with nausea and vomiting upon changes in head position.

Most severe in the lateral decubitus position with the affected ear facing down.

Persistence of vertigo for several weeks followed by its spontaneous resolution.

No hearing loss.

What is the Dix-Hallpike maneuver?

Rapid movement from a sitting to a recumbent position with the head 45° below the horizontal plane. This maneuver can induce nystagmus and vertigo. Repetition of this maneuver can attenuate the response.

Also known as Nylen-Barany test.

A 29-year-old woman complains of vertigo and diplopia. Physical examination finds that when she looks to her left, she has nystagmus of the left eye only, with failure of adduction of the right eye. The manifestation pattern of ocular motility in this case suggests the diagnosis of what disease?

Multiple sclerosis.

Internuclear ophthalmoplegia typically presents in people with multiple sclerosis. If the patient was elderly, with symptoms of new onset, the differential diagnosis would include vascular diseases.

What is the clinical presentation of idiopathic Bell palsy?

Facial weakness of the lower motor neuron type.

Pain about the ear, and may be associated with impairment of taste or lacrimation, or with hyperacusis (sensitivity to loud, low-frequency sounds).

How does Rinne test work in assessing hearing loss?

Rinne test: The base of a lightly vibrating high-pitched (512-Hz) tuning fork is placed on the mastoid process until the patient no longer perceives the sound, and the still-vibrating fork is then brought up close to (not touching) the ear.

Normal: Air conduction more rapid than bone conduction.

Sensorineural hearing loss: Air conduction more rapid than bone conduction.

Conduction hearing loss: Bone conduction more rapid than air conduction on the affected side.

What is the treatment for trigeminal neuralgia (tic douloureux)?

Carbamazepine can induce remission of symptoms in 24 hours. Phenytoin will abort an acute attack.

How does the Weber test work in assessing hearing loss?

Weber test: A high-pitched (512-Hz) tuning fork is struck and the handle placed on the midline of the patient's forehead.

Normal: Sound is perceived as coming from the midline.

Sensorineural: Sound perceived as coming from the normal ear.

Conduction hearing loss: Sound perceived as coming from the affected ear.

What is the etiology of benign positional vertigo?

Peripheral: Canalolithiasis (free-floating debris migrates into a semicircular canal and causes short episodes of vertigo when it moves within the canal).

Central: Unknown.

What are the signs of a poor prognosis in Bell palsy?

Severe pain.

Complete palsy.

What are the clinical features of diabetic ophthalmoplegia?

Isolated impairments from an isolated lesion of the oculomotor, trochlear, or abducens nerve.

Usually not detectable by brain imaging study.

Pupillary sparing: Infarction of the central portion of the oculomotor nerve with sparing of the peripheral fibers that mediate papillary regulation.

Vision may be impaired in one eye. When light is shone in the affected eye, both pupils are not reactive. When light is shone in the healthy eye, both pupils react. This pattern of reaction provides the differentiation from optic neuritis, in which the affected eye shows a diminished papillary reaction to light.

In optic neuritis, the affected eye shows a diminished pupillary reaction to light.

What are the manifestations of optic nerve pathology?

Impairment of visual acuity in one eye.

Direct and consensual responses to light are weak on the diseased side but not on the other side.

What is temporary hemianopsia and what is its most common cause?

Temporary loss of vision in one half of the visual field of one or both eyes.

Commonly caused by migraine.

CHAPTER 21 Miscellaneous Neurology Topics

What are the mechanisms of central pontine myelinolysis (CPM)?

A demyelinating disease of the central nervous system, also known as "osmotic demyelination syndrome."

Hyponatremia and its inappropriate correction are traditionally considered to be associated with CPM. However, the etiology is usually multifactorial.

Chronic alcoholism is the most common underlying disorder.

How does CPM present in imaging studies?

Computed tomography (CT): Hypodense areas within the central pons.

Magnetic resonance imaging (MRI): Hypointense on T1 and hyperintense on T2.

Of what disease is involuntary gait acceleration a characteristic feature?

Parkinson disease.

What are characteristic cerebrospinal fluid (CSF) findings in multiple sclerosis?

Oligoclonal bands of immunoglobulin G and myelin basic protein on protein electrophoresis.

What are clinical features of giant cell arteritis?

Usually elderly patients.

Severe headache associated with periods of monocular visual loss.

Aches and probable stiffness in various joints, usually in the morning.

Jaw pain is typical.

What are the clinical findings in hypertensive encephalopathy?

Systemic: A sudden increase in blood pressure may result in encephalopathy and headache in hours to days.

Gastrointestinal: Vomiting (central).

Visual disturbances, retinal arteriolar spasm, papilledema, retinal hemorrhages, and exudates.

Neurologic: Focal deficits, focal or generalized seizures.

What are common symptoms of water intoxication?

Tremor, ataxia, restlessness, diarrhea, vomiting, polyuria, and eventual stupor.

About 20% of patients with chronic schizophrenia drink water excessively, and 4% suffer from chronic hyponatremia and episodic water intoxication.

SIADH (syndrome of inappropriate secretion of antidiuretic hormone) may present with similar symptoms.

What are diagnostic tests and first-line treatment for giant cell arteritis?

Increased erythrocyte sedimentation rate.

Temporal artery biopsy.

High-dose steroids.

What are the major pathologic features of idiopathic parkinsonism?

Loss of pigmentation and cells in the substantia nigra.

Cell loss in the globus pallidus and putamen.

Presence of eosinophilic intraneural inclusion granules (Lewy bodies) in the basal ganglia, brainstem, spinal cord, and sympathetic ganglia.

Lewy bodies may appear in many forms of parkinsonism, but not in postencephalitic parkinsonism.

A patient reports involuntary jerking of the legs while falling asleep that is not associated with discomfort, and ceases during sleep. What is the likely diagnosis?

A normal phenomenon with no pathologic significance.

What are the principles of treatment for CPM?

Prevention and early diagnosis.

Correction of electrolytes at the proper rate.

Multispecialty involvement, particularly neurology.

Possible advances in use of thyroid-releasing hormone, plasmapheresis, corticosteroids, and intravenous immunoglobulins.

What are the characteristics and treatment of pseudotumor cerebri, also known as benign intracranial hypertension?

Symptoms: Headache, papilledema, and diminished visual acuity.

Evaluation: MRI or CT shows both normal and typical small, slitlike ventricles, and increased intracranial pressure.

Pseudotumor cerebri is more common in women than in men, and reaches peak frequency in the third decade.

Treatment: Acetazolamide, a carbonic anhydrase inhibitor.

What are the characteristics of cluster headache?

Quality of pain: Brief, severe, excruciating, sharp stabbing, nonthrobbing, unilateral headache, recurs on the same side, retro-orbitally, and/or in the nostril.

Time: Nighttime occurrence, awakening the patient from sleep, and may recur in the day. Duration from 10 minutes to 2 hours.

Other symptoms: Ipsilateral lacrimation, conjunctival injection, nasal stuffiness, and Horner syndrome.

Frequently occurs in men. Mean age at onset is 25 years.

What are the common findings in normal pressure hydrocephalus?

The triad of ataxia, urinary incontinence, and dementia.

Enlarged ventricles can be seen by CT or MRI.

What are the electroencephalographic (EEG) patterns of a normal sleep cycle?

Fully awake: Random fast waves;

Drowsiness: Alpha waves;

Nonrapid eye movement (NREM) stage I: Theta waves;

NREM stage II: Theta waves with sleep spindles and K complexes;

NREM stages III and IV: Delta waves;

REM: Random fast waves with sawtooth pattern.

What are the features of gait in Parkinson disease?

Postural instability and a tendency to accelerate involuntarily with small steps. The patient walks with rigid, shuffling steps and a narrow base. There is a tendency to lean forward to accelerate the speed of walking.

What are the features of giant cell arteritis?

In a typical case of giant cell arteritis, an elderly patient reports a very severe headache associated at times with periods of monocular visual loss. The patient also has aches in various joints and some stiffness in the morning. Another typical manifestation is jaw pain.

Laboratory finding: Increased erythrocyte sedimentation rate.

Diagnostic test: Temporal artery biopsy.

Treatment: High-dose steroids.

What are the first-line treatments for Wilson disease?

Avoidance of copper-rich foods.

Penicillamine.

Potassium.

Pyridoxine.

Zinc.

What are the pathologic characteristics of Wilson disease?

Psychosis and liver dysfunction.

Kayser-Fleischer ring on the cornea.

Dysarthria, tremor, poor coordination, dystonia, and hypersexuality.

What are the pros and cons of CT and MRI of the head?

CT: Economical, more widely available, the diagnostic procedure of choice for acute hemorrhage or acute trauma, suitable for those with pacemaker.

MRI: Better differentiation of white from gray matter, better identification of white matter lesions, better detection of posterior fossa and brainstem pathology, suitable for patients for whom radiation exposure is contraindicated.

What are typical imaging findings in hypertensive encephalopathy?

A CT scan or MRI T2-weighted study shows low-density areas suggestive of edema in the posterior regions of the hemispheric white matter.

What clinical findings may imply CPM?

Initial phase may look like psychiatric illness, with affective disturbances and fluctuation of consciousness.

Signs of damage in the corticobulbar and corticospinal tracts in the basis pontis, paralysis of the lower cranial nerves (pseudobulbar palsy, dysarthria, dysphagia, tetraparesis).

What does a go-no-go test evaluate?

Ask the patient to tap the underside of a table twice when the examiner taps the underside of the table once. When the examiner taps twice, the patient makes no response.

A test for frontal-subcortical system tasks.

What does a positive Romberg test imply?

Dysfunction of dorsal columns.

What is amyotrophic lateral sclerosis?

Mixed upper and lower motor neuron deficits.

Usually found in the limbs, although there may also be bulbar involvement of the upper or lower motor neuron type.

Easy fatigability, weakness, stiffness, twitching, wasting, and muscle cramping.

No sensory deficit.

Atrophy of the intrinsic muscles, brisk reflexes.

Electrophysiologic study shows widespread fasciculation, fibrillations, and positive sharp waves.

What is Brown-Sequard syndrome?

Hemisection of the spinal cord.

Ipsilateral deficit below the level of the lesion: Motor, vibration, and joint position sense.

Contralateral deficit below the level of the lesion: Loss of pain and temperature sense.

What is CPM?

A demyelinating disease of the central nervous system, also known as "osmotic demyelination syndrome."

Hyponatremia and its inappropriate correction are traditionally considered to be associated with CPM. However, the etiology is usually multifactorial.

Chronic alcoholism is the most common underlying disorder.

Initial phase may look like psychiatric illness, with affective disturbances, and fluctuation of consciousness.

Signs of damage in the corticobulbar and corticospinal tracts in the basis pontis, paralysis of the lower cranial nerves (pseudobulbar palsy, dysarthria, dysphagia, tetraparesis).

What is Guillain-Barré syndrome?

Named after two French neurologists, who among other things contributed to the initial identification of the condition.

Acute inflammatory demyelinating polyradiculoneuropathy, also known as postinfectious demyelinating polyneuropathy.

Paresthesias and numbness start in the fingers and toes, with quick involvement of feet and legs, hands, arms, and respiratory muscles, and cranial nerves.

Symptoms often follow an upper respiratory or gastrointestinal (most often *Campylobacter jejuni*) illness. Could be idiopathic.

CSF: High protein and nearly normal cell counts.

Treatment is supportive.

What is hemiballismus?

A unilateral chorea that is especially violent because the proximal muscles of the limbs are involved.

Classically attributed to vascular disease in the contralateral subthalamic nucleus. However, caudate or other basal ganglia are also believed to be associated with hemiballismus.

Possible causes include toxoplasmosis and vasculitis.

Commonly resolves spontaneously within weeks.

Dopamine-blocking agents may suppress the abnormal movements.

What is subacute combined degeneration?

Cause: Vitamin B_{12} deficiency (pernicious anemia, gastrointestinal surgery, sprue, fish tapeworm, and strict vegetarian diet).

Symptoms: Distal paresthesias, absent reflexes, weakness, loss of proprioception, spastic paraparesis, positive Babinski sign, ataxia, and dementia.

Diagnostic tests: Serum vitamin B_{12} assay, Schilling test.

What is syringomyelia?

Cavitation of the spinal cord.

Commonly occurring in the cervical region.

Dissociated sensory loss at the level of the lesion: Pinprick and temperature appreciation are impaired, but light touch and vibration sensation are preserved.

Weakness and wasting of muscles occur at the level of the lesion, and reflexes are absent.

What is the cause of benign intracranial hypertension?

The cause is unknown, but may be associated with vitamin A intoxication.

What is the characteristic EEG pattern of hepatic encephalopathy?

Large, bilaterally synchronous triphasic slow waves.

What is the clinical presentation of neurosyphilis?

Dementia and other psychiatric presentations.

CT shows generalized atrophy.

The CSF contains lymphocytes and protein. Gamma globulin is elevated.

What is the drug of choice for the treatment of psychotic symptoms in Parkinson disease?

Clozapine was once the only choice. Recent reports support olanzapine and quetiapine. The choice among these three agents should be based on clinical judgment.

What is the function of the suprachiasmatic nucleus?

The organization of behavioral and physiologic circadian rhythm.

What is the location of olfactory hallucinations followed by altered consciousness and orofacial automatisms?

Anterior medial temporal lobe.

What is the major location of subacute combined degeneration of the spinal cord in pernicious anemia?

Posterior and lateral funiculi.

What is the mechanism of action of carbidopa in the treatment of Parkinson disease?

Blockade of peripheral dopa decarboxylase, augmenting the action of levodopa.

What is the most important condition to be considered in a senile patient with headaches and pain in the jaw muscles when chewing?

Temporal arteritis.

What is the neuropathologic hallmark of Marchiafava-Bignami disease?

Atrophy and demyelination of the corpus callosum.

Marchiafava-Bignami disease occurs most often in malnourished alcoholics.

The clinical features are dementia, spasticity, dysarthria, and gait disturbance.

What is the treatment of choice for nocturnal myoclonic sleep disorder?

Benzodiazepines.

What is the treatment of choice for the abnormal involuntary movement associated with Huntington chorea?

Haloperidol, chlorpromazine, or reserpine (a dopamine-depleting agent).

Huntington chorea:

Typical features: Dementia and chorea, with a positive family history.

Molecular mechanism: Expansion of CAG trinucleotide repeat sequences at chromosome 4p16.3.

What is the type of tremor characteristic of Parkinson disease?

Rest tremor, or tremor that is prominent in the resting state, and attenuated during voluntary movement (e.g., when the patient attempts to do the finger-nose-finger test).

What pharmacologic treatments are used for migraine?

Acute treatment: Nonnarcotic analgesics, prochlorperazine, ergotamine, dihydroergotamine, and sumatriptan (Imitrex).

Prophylaxis: Tricyclic antidepressants (amitriptyline, nortriptyline), low-dose ergot preparations, methysergide, valproate, calcium channel antagonists (verapamil, nifedipine).

What vitamin, taken before conception, can reduce the incidence of neural tube defects?

Folic acid.

It is recommended that pregnant female patients who take valproic acid take folic acid.

Where is the site of pathology for Klüver-Bucy syndrome?

Amygdaloid nucleus.

APPENDIX I Board-Type Questions and Answers

1. An adolescent girl cleans her room meticulously after a heated argument with her mother about her miniskirt. What defense mechanism is most likely associated with her behavior?

A. Displacement.
B. Projection.
C. Idealization.
D. Sublimation.
E. Splitting.

The answer is D.

Sublimation is the channeling of unacceptable impulses into more acceptable outlets.

Displacement is the redirecting of thoughts, feelings, and impulses from an object that gives rise to anxiety to a safer, more acceptable one. Example: Being angry at the boss and kicking the dog.

Projection is the attribution of one's undesired impulses onto another. Example: An angry party of an argument accuses the other party of hostility.

Idealization is the overestimation of the desirable qualities and underestimation of the limitations of a desired object. Example: A lover speaks in glowing terms of (and consciously believes) the intelligence of a woman who is not very bright.

Splitting is a primitive defense mechanism in which a person sees external objects or people as either "all good" or "all bad."

2. A 67-year-old senior manager came to your office with complaints of forgetfulness and difficulty in working on his company's electronic data system. This has gradually become worse in the past year. He worries that he may have to retire soon, though he really would like to continue to work until his 70th birthday. He denies other stresses. He denies significant mood disturbance besides mild to moderate anxiety about his ability to work. He has no previous psychiatric history. To clarify the diagnosis, you decided to order some lab tests and a psychometric test. Which of the following is the most appropriate test?

A. Rorschach test.
B. Wisconsin Card Sorting Test.
C. Brief Psychotic Rating Scale.
D. Minnesota Multiphasic Personality Inventory-2.
E. Millon Clinical Multiaxial Inventory-2.

The answer is B.

The case demands a cognitive test. Among the listed tests, only the Wisconsin Card Sorting Test is a cognitive test. Rorschach is a projective test designed to detect the presence of subtle psychotic thought processes and bizarre ideation. Brief Psychotic Rating Scale is a quantitative scale for psychotic symptoms. Minnesota Multiphasic Personality Inventory-2 and Millon Clinical Multiaxial Inventory-2 are tools for assessment of personality traits.

3. The following are symptoms of complicated bereavement EXCEPT:

A. Guilt.
B. Suicidal ideation.
C. Anger toward God.
D. Psychomotor retardation.
E. Preoccupation with worthlessness.

The answer is C.

Symptoms that imply complication of major depression are: Suicidal ideation, guilt, psychomotor retardation, hallucination, preoccupation with worthlessness, and symptoms lasting longer than 2 months.

Extreme sadness, crying spells, and anger toward God are symptoms of uncomplicated bereavement.

4. A 52-year-old white man was admitted for depression comorbid with severe alcohol withdrawal subsequent to recurrent intoxication. His hepatic enzymes were moderately elevated. As his psychiatrist, you decided to start the treatment with detoxification using the proper benzodiazepine. Though chlordiazepoxide is used in your regular detoxification protocol, you decided to use lorazepam in this case. This is because lorazepam does not require which metabolic reaction that an impaired liver may not able to process efficiently?

A. Oxidation.
B. Conjugation.
C. Absorption.
D. Acetylation.
E. Glucuronidation.

The answer is A.

The two major processes of liver metabolism are oxidation and conjugation. Oxidation heavily relies on liver enzymes, while conjugation may happen with or without liver enzymes. Therefore in patients with severe liver impairment, medicines that require oxidation are not appropriate. There are three benzodiazepines that require no oxidation: Temazepam, oxazepam, and lorazepam. Absorption is not directly influenced by liver function. Acetylation may happen outside of the liver. Glucuronidation is one of the conjugation reactions.

5. At what age do children start to understand that death is permanent?

A. 1 year.
B. 3 years.
C. 5 years.
D. 7 years.
E. 9 years.

The answer is D.

At the age of 7 children start to understand that death is permanent.

6. In patients with anxiety disorders, the following are risk factors implying a possible organic etiology EXCEPT:

A. Onset after 25.
B. Lack of familial history of anxiety disorders.
C. No significant triggering events.
D. Lack of avoidance behavior.
E. Poor response to anxiolytic agents.

The answer is A.

Onset after 40 is a factor that implies organic etiology for anxiety disorders.

7. A 70-year-old man presents with progressive dementia. A magnetic resonance imaging (MRI) scan shows multiple areas of increased T2-weighted density in the periventricular area. What is the most likely diagnosis?

A. Pseudotumor cerebri.
B. Normal-pressure hydrocephalus.
C. Multi-infarct dementia.
D. Pick's disease.
E. Metastatic carcinoma.

The answer is C.

The MRI finding is pathognomonic for multi-infarct dementia.

Pseudotumor cerebri: MRI shows small ventricles.

Normal-pressure hydrocephalus: MRI shows enlarged lateral ventricles.

Pick's disease: MRI shows frontal- and temporal-lobe atrophy.

Metastatic carcinoma: MRI shows multiple coinlike lesions.

8. Neuroleptic malignant syndrome (NMS) commonly presents with each of the following EXCEPT:

A. Elevated creatine kinase.
B. Rigidity and tremor.
C. Leukopenia.
D. Labile blood pressure.
E. Fever.

The answer is C.

NMS is usually associated with leukocytosis, not leukopenia.

9. Focal dystonia (blepharospasm, oromandibular dystonia, spasmodic torticollis, writer's cramp, etc.) can be effectively treated with:

A. Haloperidol.
B. Reserpine.
C. Surgical denervation.
D. Botulinum toxin.
E. Baclofen.

The answer is D.

Haloperidol, an antipsychotic agent, can be used in the treatment of Gilles de la Tourette syndrome.

Baclofen is a centrally acting muscle relaxant and can be used in the treatment of trigeminal neuralgia and other painful spasms. It is not an effective treatment for focal dystonia.

Reserpine and surgical denervation are not usually used in treating focal dystonia.

10. A 25-year-old man complains of recurrent severe headache. He states that his headache usually occurs in the early morning. Sometimes he was awakened by the headache. The pain lasts from 30 to 60 minutes. It is excruciating and stabbing. The pain begins at his left nostril, and this is followed by severe retro-orbital pain. It is accompanied by tearing and nasal stuffiness on the left side of the face. The patient's

mother, who has witnessed his episodes, has noted injection of his left eye and swelling of the left side of his face during the headache. The most likely diagnosis is:

A. Giant cell arteritis.
B. Trigeminal neuralgia.
C. Migraine.
D. Cluster headache.
E. Glaucoma.

The answer is D.

Giant cell arteritis is seen primarily in the elderly. The onset is abrupt or insidious over a period of weeks. Typical symptoms include unilateral headache involving the jaw, tongue, and temporal region, and visual disturbances. Eye injection and facial swelling are not associated with this condition.

Trigeminal neuralgia produces severe pain in the distribution of one or more of the divisions of the trigeminal nerve, most commonly the second or third division. Symptoms rarely present at night. The pain may be elicited by tickle or touch. The pain usually occurs in bursts lasting several seconds, which are followed by a refractory period.

Migraine is a paroxysmal headache lasting for hours to days, with or without an aura. The pain is usually unilateral, throbbing, and intensified by movement. Sleep may abort the pain.

Glaucoma presents with a dull ache in or around one eye, with mildly blurred vision and halos around lights. Symptoms occur when watching television or reading in a dark room.

11. All of the following occur in normal pressure hydrocephalus EXCEPT:

A. Gait disturbance (ataxia).
B. Enlarged ventricles.
C. Urinary incontinence.
D. Dementia.
E. Positive Romberg sign.

The answer is E.

A positive Romberg sign usually presents in spinal conditions.

12. A left-handed woman had a recent cerebrovascular accident. She is able to comprehend and follow commands. However, she is unable to speak with correct grammar, and cannot repeat other people's words. Her speech is nonfluent and telegraphic. All of the following are correct EXCEPT:

A. This patient most likely also has a visual field reduction.
B. This is a case of Broca aphasia.
C. The cerebral lesion involves the left frontal lobe.
D. The patient most likely also has right hemiparesis.
E. The patient's type of aphasia is also known as expressive aphasia.

The answer is A.

A visual field reduction is a symptom associated with disturbance in the optic tract, optic chiasm, or optic nerve, and not with a cortical disturbance. Broca area is not associated with visual function.

In the majority (80%) of left-handed people, the left cerebrum is the dominant side.

13. The following are contraindicated for concomitant use with monoamine oxidase inhibitors (MAOIs) EXCEPT:

A. Meperidine.
B. Aged cheese.
C. Phentolamine.
D. Phenylephrine.
E. Fluoxetine.

The answer is C.

Phentolamine is an α-adrenergic antagonist that may be used to treat MAOI-related hypertensive crises.

14. Which of the following is NOT a characteristic feature of complex partial seizures?

A. A commonly associated symptom is an epigastric sensation.
B. Affect is usually flattened.
C. Consciousness is impaired but not lost.
D. Olfactory hallucinations and déjà vu may appear.
E. The majority of patients present with automatism.

The answer is B.

Complex partial seizures are associated with intensified affect.

15. A 30-year-old woman complains of severe headaches and episodes of brief loss of vision. She states that she has been depressed and has gained 50 pounds in the past 12 months. A neurologic examination yields insignificant findings except for bilateral papilledema. An MRI scan of the brain shows small ventricles. Lumbar puncture reveals elevated cerebrospinal fluid (CSF) pressure. What is the most likely diagnosis?

A. Pseudotumor cerebri.
B. Normal pressure hydrocephalus.
C. Major depressive disorder (MDD).
D. Bacterial meningitis.
E. Metastatic carcinoma.

The answer is A.

Normal pressure hydrocephalus: MRI shows enlarged lateral ventricles. CSF pressure is not elevated.

MDD: No significant neurologic effect.

Meningitis: Usually no change in the MRI.

Metastatic carcinoma: Typical MRI finding is multiple coinlike lesions.

16. A 35-year-old woman suffers from progressive dementia and involuntary dancelike movements. She has a positive family history of these same manifestations. Genetic study reports an expansion of CAG trinucleotide repeat sequences at chromosome 4p16.3. Which of the following agents is the best treatment for the patient's abnormal involuntary movements?

A. Benztropine.
B. Haloperidol.
C. L-Dihydroxyphenylalanine (L-dopa).
D. Stereotactic thalamotomy.
E. Lorazepam.

The answer is B.

This is a typical case of Huntington disease. Haloperidol is the treatment of choice.

Benztropine is a treatment for drug-induced parkinsonism.

L-dopa is a treatment for Parkinson disease.

Stereotactic thalamotomy is a treatment for intractable seizure.

Lorazepam is used in a variety of disorders. Its intravenous (IV) form is particularly useful for aborting seizures. It is not effective for Huntington disease.

17. In older populations, drug metabolism is changed by the following factor(s):

A. Decrease in body fat.
B. Increased perfusion of the liver.
C. Increased plasma-binding proteins.
D. Increased renal clearance.
E. Decreased hepatic metabolism.

The answer is E.

The metabolic change in elderly persons is in the opposite direction from all of the listed statements except E.

18. A 49-year-old man experiences progressive weakness for several months. He also complains of muscle twitching, cramps, easy fatigability, and stiffness in his arms and legs. Physical examination shows atrophy of the intrinsic muscles, and the reflexes are brisk. There are no sensory findings. Electrophysiologic study shows widespread fasciculations, fibrillation, and positive sharp waves. The history and results of examinations strongly suggest which of the following diagnoses?

A. Multiple sclerosis.
B. Fascioscapulohumeral muscular dystrophy.
C. Amyotrophic lateral sclerosis.
D. Chronic fatigue syndrome.
E. Myasthenia gravis.

The answer is C.

Multiple sclerosis: Involves different parts of the central nervous system (CNS). Symptoms are often transient, disappearing after a few days or weeks. They may include changes in vision and disturbances in bladder function. Sensory deficits may appear. Diagnosis is based on the clinical picture, CSF findings (oligoclonal bands), MRI, and other tests.

Fascioscapulohumeral muscular dystrophy: Rearrangement of a homeobox gene on the long arm of chromosome 4. Onset in adolescence. Weakness is confined to the face, neck, and shoulder.

Chronic fatigue syndrome should not have any neurologic signs.

Myasthenia gravis: Impaired neuromuscular transmission. Most cases involve extraocular muscles. Sustained activity of affected muscles leads to temporarily increased weakness. Sensation is normal. No reflex changes. Electrophysiologic testing shows decremental responses of muscle to repetitive supramaximal stimulation of the muscle motor nerve, but normal findings are also possible.

19. A 39-year-old woman experiences progressive weakness of her arms and legs over a period of several days. Physical examination reveals symmetric weakness and absence of deep tendon reflexes. CSF testing shows an elevated protein with 6 lymphocytes/mm^3. Nerve conduction study reports show a slow conduction velocity, prolonged distal motor latency, and conduction block. What is the most likely diagnosis?

A. Polymyositis.
B. Guillain-Barré syndrome
C. Myasthenia gravis.
D. Normal pressure hydrocephalus.
E. Amyotrophic lateral sclerosis.

The answer is B.

Polymyositis: Rare in developed countries. Weakness is accompanied by myalgia and signs of meningeal irritation, and is asymmetric in distribution. Diagnosis is based on the isolation of the virus from the stool and/or nasopharyngeal secretions, and less commonly from the CSF.

Myasthenia gravis: Impaired neuromuscular transmission. Most cases involve extraocular muscles. Sustained activity of affected muscles leads to temporarily increased weakness. Sensation is normal. No changes in reflexes. Electrophysiologic testing shows decremental responses of muscle to repetitive supramaximal stimulation of the muscle motor nerve, but normal findings are also possible.

Normal pressure hydrocephalus: MRI shows enlarged lateral ventricles. No elevated CSF pressure. No change in nerve conduction.

Amyotrophic lateral sclerosis: Mixed upper and lower motor neuron deficit. No change in nerve conduction. No abnormalities in CSF tests.

20. The following are effective treatments for obsessive-compulsive disorder EXCEPT:

A. Paroxetine 50 mg per day.
B. Clomipramine 250 mg per day.
C. Phenelzine 15 mg three times a day.
D. Fluoxetine 20 mg per day.
E. Fluvoxamine 150 mg twice a day.

The answer is D.

The treatment of obsessive-compulsive disorder requires a high-dose antidepressant with a serotonergic effect.

21. Neurologic examination of a 72-year-old man reveals postural instability and a tendency to accelerate involuntarily with small steps. The patient walks with rigid, shuffling steps and a narrow base. There is a tendency to lean forward to accelerate the speed of walking. The clinical presentation is typical for:

A. Sensory ataxia.
B. Alcoholic cerebellar degeneration.
C. Normal aging.
D. Huntington chorea.
E. Parkinson disease.

The answer is E.

Sensory ataxia: A syndrome that may be caused by polyneuropathy and myelopathy. Impaired proprioceptive sensation exists at all levels of the sensory pathway. Defective joint position, a positive Romberg sign, and a slapping or steppage gait are typical symptoms of sensory ataxia.

Alcoholic cerebellar degeneration: Usually restricted to the superior vermis. Gait ataxia, distal sensory deficits in the feet, and absent ankle reflexes are common symptoms.

Normal aging may be associated with general weakness and slowness, but not with the typical parkinsonian symptoms described above.

Huntington chorea: Typical onset is between 30 and 50 years of age. The condition terminates fatally 10 to 20 years after clinical onset. Chorea is manifested as dancelike gross movements. In the early stage of the disease, fidgeting or restlessness may appear. Diagnosis is based on genetic testing, which shows expanded CAG trinucleotide repeat sequences in the short arm of chromosome 4.

22. Indications for psychostimulants are all of the following EXCEPT:

A. Attention-deficit/hyperactivity disorder (ADHD).
B. Personality disorders.
C. Narcolepsy.
D. Exogenous obesity.
E. Depression in elderly and medically ill patients.

The answer is B.

Psychostimulants should not be used in personality disorders or for patients with a history of substance abuse.

23. A 43-year-old woman complains of recurrent episodes of severe vertigo with nausea and vomiting. The symptoms usually occur with a change in head position, and are most severe in the lateral decubitus position with the left ear facing down. Neurologic examination reveals left-sided nystagmus before the occurrence of symptoms when the patient is moved from a sitting to a recumbent position. Upon repeated positional testing, the patient's symptoms are found to become less severe. Her hearing is normal. Neurologic examination is otherwise insignificant. The most likely diagnosis is:

A. Ménière disease.
B. Basilar artery insufficiency.
C. Orthostatic hypotension.
D. Cerebellar infarct.
E. Benign positional vertigo.

The answer is E.

Ménière disease: Vertigo is not associated with changes in head position. Hearing deteriorates in Ménière disease.

Basilar artery insufficiency: Although the auditory nerve is supplied by a branch of the basilar artery, basilar artery insufficiency usually involves many other structures, and always involves the dorsal portion of the pons. It causes abducens nerve palsy, impaired horizontal eye movements, and vertical nystagmus. Hemiplegia or quadriplegia is usually present, and coma is common.

Orthostatic hypotension: Dizziness, lightheadedness, but no vertigo.

Cerebellar infarct: Coma of acute onset, and rapid deterioration that leads to death.

24. Electroconvulsive therapy (ECT) is likely to be effective for the following conditions EXCEPT:

A. Catatonia.
B. Delirium.
C. Acute mania.
D. Severe depression.
E. Somatization disorder.

The answer is E.

ECT is not effective in somatization disorder, personality disorders, or anxiety disorders.

25. A 40-year-old woman complains of persistent numbness on the palmar surface of her right hand, and of pain in her right arm. Her symptoms are more severe in the morning. Neurologic examination reveals a sensory deficit in the right thumb, index, and middle fingers, as well as on the lateral half of the ring finger. The patient has weakness in abducting the thumb. Laboratory tests reveal an elevated level of thyroid-stimulating hormone. Which of the following is the most likely diagnosis?

A. Ulnar nerve entrapment.
B. Radial nerve compression.
C. Carpal tunnel syndrome.
D. Radial fracture.
E. Atherosclerosis.

The answer is C.

Ulnar nerve entrapment impairs adduction of the little finger. There is a sensory deficit on the palmar surface and back of the little finger and on the lateral side of the ring finger.

Radial nerve compression: Difficulty in adducting (not abducting) the thumb. There is a sensory deficit on the back of the hand between the thumb and index finger.

Radial fracture: May be associated with radial nerve damage.

Atherosclerosis: No typical distribution of deficits as described in this case.

26. Many drugs may change the serum lithium level. In the following list, the drug that may decrease the serum lithium level is:

A. Nonsteroidal anti-inflammatory drug.
B. Ibuprofen.
C. Indomethacin.
D. Theophylline.
E. Spironolactone.

The answer is D.

Theophylline is the only one of the drugs listed that may decrease the serum lithium level. All of the remaining drugs may increase serum lithium levels.

27. Which of the following medicines is associated with the development of ataxia, gingival hyperplasia, hirsutism, agranulocytosis, and coarse facial features?

A. Phenytoin.
B. Carbamazepine.
C. Valproic acid.
D. Topiramate.
E. Oxcarbazepine.

The answer is A.

Ataxia, although it has a neurologic definition, may be clinically difficult to differentiate from many forms of gait unsteadiness, and therefore is too general a term to point to a specific drug.

Gingival hyperplasia is a specific reaction to phenytoin. Another anticonvulsant that may have a similar reaction is ethosuximide.

Many drugs may promote extra hair growth. Phenytoin is a well-known such drug. Valproic acid may cause hair loss. Carbamazepine and topiramate are not associated with hirsutism.

Hirsutism in oxcarbazepine users is rare.

Agranulocytosis is associated with many drugs. Of the drugs listed, only topiramate is not associated with bone-marrow suppression.

28. A 9-year-old boy is observed to have several episodes of brief "out-of-mind" spells. His family notices that in such spells he suddenly stops his activities, blinks his eyes, and turns his head to the left. Each spell lasts a couple of seconds. The boy never falls during these spells, and recovers completely to a normal state. What is the appropriate treatment for this boy?

A. Carbamazepine.
B. Valproic acid.
C. Lamotrigine.
D. Gabapentin.
E. Phenytoin.

The answer is B.

This boy suffers from absence seizures, also known as petit mal seizures. Treatment consists of ethosuximide and valproic acid.

29. In order to obtain therapeutic effect from ECT, which of the following is required?

A. Loss of consciousness.
B. Electrical stimulation of the left hemisphere.
C. Bilateral spread of convulsion.
D. Induction of amnesia.
E. Anesthesia.

The answer is C.

Bilateral convulsion is the only one of the foregoing conditions in which there is consistent evidence of a therapeutic effect of ECT.

30. All of the following are choices of pharmacologic treatment in ADHD EXCEPT:

A. Methylphenidate.
B. Bupropion.
C. Clonidine.
D. Propranolol.
E. Pemoline.

The answer is D.

Choices for treatment of ADHD are stimulants, antidepressants, and clonidine.

31. What is the treatment of choice for lithium-induced polyuria and polydipsia?

A. Reduce fluid intake.
B. Amiloride.
C. Propranolol.
D. Mannitol.
E. Furosemide.

The answer is B.

Lithium inhibits free-water resorption at the collecting tubule. Amiloride is a potassium-sparing diuretic that inhibits sodium resorption at the distal convoluted tubule. Amiloride can reduce the symptoms of polyuria and polydipsia.

Reducing fluid intake, mannitol, and furosemide worsen the symptoms of lithium-induced polyuria and polydipsia. Propranolol is useful in treating lithium-induced tremor, not polyuria/polydipsia.

32. What is the most common side effect of clozapine?

A. Seizure.
B. Agranulocytosis.
C. Hypotension.
D. Sedation.
E. Increased prolactin level.

The answer is D.

Seizure and agranulocytosis are both rare but severe, and hence notorious, adverse reactions to clozapine. Clozapine may cause hypotension, but the most common side effect is sedation. Clozapine has minimal effect on serum prolactin levels, which is one of the features that make it the gold standard of atypical antipsychotic agents.

33. Which of the following is not a symptom of serotonin syndrome?

A. Jitteriness and tremor.
B. Hypotension.
C. Hypotonicity.
D. Diaphoresis.
E. Hypertension.

The answer is C.

Hypertonicity may appear in serotonin syndrome.

Autonomic instability is one of the key features of serotonin syndrome. It may present with either hypo- or hypertension.

34. Mirtazapine is a unique antidepressant that blocks the following receptors EXCEPT:

A. Type 1 histamine receptor (H1).
B. α_2-Adrenergic receptor (α_2).
C. Type 1 serotonin receptor (5-HT_1).
D. Type 2 serotonin receptor (5-HT_2).
E. Type 3 serotonin receptor (5-HT_3).

The answer is C.

Mirtazapine blocks central α_2-adrenergic receptors and increases serotonergic tone. It blocks 5-HT_2 and 5-HT_3 receptors, reducing anxiety and gastrointestinal reactivity, and enhances serotonergic binding to 5-HT_{1a} and 5-HT_{1c} receptors. Mirtazapine also blocks H1 receptors, which gives mirtazapine its sedative effect.

35. Bupropion is contraindicated in patients with:

A. Myocardial infarction.
B. Alcohol dependence.
C. Obesity.
D. Sexual dysfunction.
E. Eating disorder.

The answer is E.

Another important contraindication to bupropion is seizure disorder.

Bupropion is not contraindicated in cardiac conditions or in alcohol/drug dependence. Bupropion may reduce sexual dysfunction induced by selective serotonin reuptake inhibitors (SSRIs), and even improves sexual function in some cases. One of the side effects of bupropion is weight loss.

36. The reaction to anticipated death, according to Elizabeth Kübler-Ross, includes which of the following orders of stages?

A. Denial, anger, bargaining, depression, and acceptance.
B. Denial, shock, anger, bargaining, and acceptance.
C. Denial, depression, bargaining, anger, and acceptance.
D. Shock, anger, bargaining, acceptance, and gratefulness.
E. Denial, rumination, bargaining, anger, and acceptance.

The answer is A.

1. Shock and denial.
2. Anger.
3. Bargaining.
4. Depression.
5. Acceptance.

37. The characteristic features of Rett disorder are the following EXCEPT:

A. Deceleration of head growth beginning in early childhood.
B. Macro-orchidism.
C. Loss of previously acquired purposeful hand skills.
D. Loss of social engagement.
E. Severely impaired language development.

The answer is B.

Macro-orchidism is a feature of fragile X syndrome, not of Rett disorder.

38. According to Erik Erikson, the developmental crisis most typical of normal teenagers involves:

A. Initiative versus guilt.
B. Intimacy versus isolation.
C. Ego integrity versus despair.
D. Identity versus role confusion.
E. Autonomy versus shame and doubt.

The answer is D.

Basic trust versus mistrust: Age 0 to 1 year.

Autonomy versus shame and doubt: Age 1 to 3 years.

Initiative versus guilt: Age 3 to 6 years.

Industry versus inferiority: Age 6 to 12 years.

Identity versus role confusion: Age 12 to 20 years.

Intimacy versus isolation: Age 20 to 40 years.

Generativity versus stagnation: Age 40 to 65 years.

Ego integrity versus despair: Age 65 years and older.

39. Orthostatic hypotension and priapism are associated with which of the following effects?

A. α_1-Adrenergic receptor stimulation.
B. α_1-Adrenergic receptor blockade.
C. α_2-Adrenergic receptor stimulation.
D. α_2-Adrenergic receptor blockade.
E. Muscarinic cholinergic receptor blockade.

The answer is B.

α_1-Adrenergic receptor stimulation may cause vascular contraction, and result in elevation of blood pressure.

α_2-Adrenergic receptor is a presynaptic receptor. Stimulation of α_2-adrenergic receptors may cause decreased release of norepinephrine and serotonin (e.g., as with clonidine). Blockade of α_2-adrenergic receptors increases the release of norepinephrine and serotonin (e.g., as with mirtazapine).

An anticholinergic effect may cause dizziness and drowsiness, which is similar to what occurs with α_1-adrenergic receptor blockade. However, cholinergic receptors do not have a direct effect on vascular activity.

40. Adverse effects of lithium include the following EXCEPT:

A. Tremor.
B. Nephrogenic diabetes insipidus.
C. Weight gain.
D. Hypothyroidism.
E. Exacerbation of narrow-angle glaucoma.

The answer is E.

An anticholinergic effect is associated with exacerbation of narrow-angle glaucoma. Lithium does not have an anticholinergic effect.

41. The following are associated with the effect of venlafaxine, EXCEPT:

A. Blockade of serotonin reuptake.
B. Blockade of norepinephrine reuptake.
C. Blockade of dopamine reuptake.
D. Possibly elevated systolic but not diastolic blood pressure.
E. No significant inhibition of cytochrome P450.

The answer is D.

Venlafaxine mainly causes elevated diastolic blood pressure.

42. The "learned helplessness" animal model is proposed for the research of which of the following psychiatric illnesses?

A. Schizophrenia.
B. Anxiety.
C. Depression.
D. Mania.
E. Aggression.

The answer is C.

"Learned helplessness" is one of the many animal models for the study of depression. Others include pharmacologic models (e.g., the reserpine syndrome model); separation models (maternal separation or peer separation); and chronic stress models, as well as others.

Drug-related (amphetamine, phencyclidine, and hallucinogen) animal models and sensorimotor-gating models of schizophrenia are commonly applied to schizophrenia research.

Operant conditioning paradigms are usually used to establish animal models for the study of anxiety.

For mania and aggression, there is so far no commonly used animal model.

43. What method of producing a stimulus could make an experimental animal most resistant to extinction?

A. A fixed-interval schedule.
B. A fixed-ratio schedule.
C. A variable-ratio schedule.
D. Positive reinforcement.

The answer is C.

The most difficult way to extinguish a stimulus is to produce it on a variable-ratio schedule, or in an intermittent, relatively unpredictable fashion. The fixed-ratio schedule causes habituation but not resistance to extinction. Positive reinforcement is necessary for creating resistance to extinction, but the means of delivery of the stimulus is more important. Consider a mediocre researcher who occasionally gets a paper published and gets low-level grants once every few years. It is very hard for such a person to give up his or her effort because reinforcement provided is on a variable-ratio schedule!

44. A 2-year-old boy has strong attachment to his parents. What will be his reaction when he sees his parents return to the room in which he is present after a brief separation from him?

A. Continued play.
B. Brief contact followed by continued play.
C. Intense anger.
D. Sustained contact and cessation of play.
E. Avoidance of the parents.

The answer is B.

Based on Mary Ainsworth's study, more than 60% of children develop secure attachments by the age of 24 months. Attachment is the bonding that develops between a child and its primary caregiver. Children usually consider their primary caregiver as the symbol of security and resources available to them.

In this case, the typical reaction of the child is brief contact followed by continued play.

45. Applying positive and negative stimuli to alter the frequency of behavior is called:

A. Classical conditioning.
B. Operant conditioning.
C. Partial reinforcement.
D. Respondent learning.
E. Higher-order conditioning.

The answer is B.

Also known as instrumental conditioning, operant conditioning is a form of learning in which behavioral frequency is altered through the application of positive and negative consequences. B.F. Skinner developed the theory of operant conditioning. As an example of such conditioning, a dog might receive food only when it correctly responds by pressing a lever. Food is the reinforcing stimulus and the lever is the operant.

Classical conditioning, developed by Ivan Pavlov, results from the repeated pairing of a neutral (conditioned) stimulus with one that evokes a response (unconditioned stimulus), such that the neutral stimulus eventually comes to evoke the response. This is also called respondent learning. The establishing of a new conditioned stimulus through coupling with an established stimulus is called higher-order conditioning.

Partial reinforcement means that reinforcement of a particular behavior occurs intermittently. This makes the behavior highly resistant to extinction.

46. Based on Sigmund Freud's theory, what does a 4-year-old boy fear?

A. Castration by his father.
B. Aggression toward his mother.
C. Death of his father.
D. Identification with his father.

The answer is A.

This boy is in his phallic phase and could have castration anxiety. Another possible presentation could be an Oedipus complex.

The other items in the question are confusing.

Sigmund Freud's stages of psychosexual development are:

1. Oral (birth to 18 months).
2. Anal (1 to 3 years).
3. Phallic (oedipal, 3 to 5 years).
4. Latency (5 to 12 years).
5. Genital (12 years to adulthood).

47. What is the Wisconsin Card Sorting Test indicated to evaluate?

A. Malingering.
B. Visual-spatial memory.
C. Attention.
D. Executive functions.

The answer is D.

In the Wisconsin Card Sorting Test (WCST), the test-taker is required to match his response cards to the stimulus card by following certain rules (such as color, form, and number). The rules change without notification of the test-taker, but the correct response is learned by feedback. The test-taker needs to recognize the current rules and follow them in the card-playing process. In this way, the test-taker's executive function is examined.

The best test for detecting malingering is the clinical interview. The neuropsychologic test that helps in this regard is the Minnesota Multiphasic Personality Inventory (MMPI).

Visual-spatial memory is tested with the Rey-Osterrieth Complex Figure test or Draw-a-Clock-Face test.

Attention and concentration are tested with the Digit Span test of the Wechsler Adult Intelligence Scale-III (WAIS-III) or with the Trail-Making test Parts A and B.

48. All of the following are projective tests EXCEPT:

A. Rorschach test.
B. Thematic apperception test.
C. Sentence completion test.
D. MMPI.
E. Draw-a-Person Test.

The answer is D.

The MMPI is not a projective test.

The remaining projective tests can detect subtle psychotic thought processes and bizarre ideation.

49. What does the comprehension subtest of the WAIS measure?

A. Attention and concentration.
B. Receptive and expressive language.
C. Ability to abstract.
D. Memory function.

The answer is C.

In WAIS-III:

The comprehension subtest measures executive functions and abstract thinking.

The mental control subtest of the Wechsler Memory Scale-III (WMS-III) and WAIS-III Digit Span test measure attention and concentration.

The Verbal Intelligence Quotient subtest measures receptive and expressive language function.

The WMS-III measures memory function.

WAIS-III itself measures adult (16 to 89 years) general intelligence. The Wechsler Preschool and Primary Scale of Intelligence is for children aged

4 to 6 years. The Wechsler Intelligence Scale for Children-III is for children aged 5 to 16 years. Three major IQ test-score components are: Full-scale IQ, Verbal IQ, and Performance IQ.

50. Researchers conduct a study by following a group of subjects chosen from a well-defined population over a period of time. This type of study is a:

A. Cohort study.
B. Cross-sectional study.
C. Case-control study.
D. Case-history study.
E. Retrospective study.

The answer is A.

Cohort study (also known as follow-up study): A group of individuals (cohort) is defined on the basis of the presence or absence of exposure to a suspected risk factor for a disease, and is followed for an extended period. A cohort study is a form of prospective study.

Case-control study: Subjects are selected on the basis of whether they do or do not have a particular disease being studied.

51. What is the term for the relative frequency of a condition in a population as measured at a particular point in time?

A. Sensitivity.
B. Specificity.
C. Incidence.
D. Prevalence.

The answer is D.

Prevalence is the proportion of individuals with existing disease at a point in time (point prevalence) or during a period of time (period prevalence). It refers to all persons who are diseased within a given population.

Incidence is the proportion of individuals developing new disease during a period of time. It refers only to new cases of disease.

Sensitivity measures the ability of a test to identify true-positive cases of disease. Specificity measures the ability of a test to identify true-negative cases of the disease.

52. You encourage your patient to stop smoking so as to reduce the patient's risk of getting lung cancer. Which type of prevention is this?

A. Primary prevention.
B. Secondary prevention.
C. Tertiary prevention.
D. Not prevention, just a suggestion.

The answer is A.

Primary prevention: To prevent the onset of a disease and thereby reduce its incidence by eliminating the causative agents, reducing risk factors, enhancing host resistance, and interfering with disease transmission.

Secondary prevention: Early identification and prompt treatment of an illness, with the goal of reducing the prevalence of the condition by reducing its duration.

Tertiary prevention: Reducing the prevalence of residual defects and disabilities caused by an illness. This enables persons with chronic mental illnesses to reach the highest feasible level of function.

53. You recommend vocational therapy to your schizophrenia patients after they have been stable for some period of time. Which type of prevention is this?

A. Primary prevention.
B. Secondary prevention.
C. Tertiary prevention.
D. Not prevention, just a recommendation.

The answer is C.

Please do not make a mistake on this topic. Read the above answer for reference.

54. A social worker helps psychiatric patients obtain the services already available from the community. Which kind of service model is this?

A. Assertive community treatment.
B. Traditional social work.
C. Both.
D. Neither.

The answer is B.

Assertive community treatment: Active outreach to patients.

Traditional social work: Helps patients connect to existing services.

55. What is the most common cause of death among male African American youths?

A. Suicide.
B. Homicide.
C. Traffic accident.
D. Substance abuse.

The answer is B.

Homicide is the most common cause of death among young African American males.

56. The major inhibitory neurotransmitter in the CNS is:

A. Glutamate.
B. γ-Aminobutyric acid (GABA).
C. Dopamine.
D. Serotonin.

The answer is B.

GABA is the major inhibitory neurotransmitter in the CNS. Glycine is the major inhibitory neurotransmitter in the brainstem and peripheral nervous system (PNS). Glutamate is the major excitatory neurotransmitter in the CNS and PNS. Both dopamine and serotonin are regulatory neurotransmitters.

57. The cell bodies of which type of neuron are located in the ventral tegmental area (VTA)?

A. Dopaminergic.
B. Serotonergic.
C. Noradrenergic.
D. GABAergic.

The answer is A.

1. Dopaminergic: Three locations.
   A. Substantia nigra (nigrostriatal pathway, associated with extrapyramidal syndromes [EPS]).
   B. VTA, mesolimbic-mesocortical pathway associated with antipsychotic effects, and reward system.
   C. Hypothalamus, including the arcuate and periventricular nuclei (tuberoinfundibular pathway, associated with prolactin regulation).
2. Serotonergic:
   A. Raphe nuclei (upper pons and midbrain).
   B. Caudal locus ceruleus (to a lesser extent).
3. Noradrenergic: Locus ceuleus (pons).
4. GABAergic: GABAergic neurons are small interneurons prevalent throughout the CNS.

58. Of which hormone has dopamine been shown to inhibit the release?

A. Thyroid-stimulating hormone.
B. Follicle-stimulating hormone.
C. Luteinizing hormone.
D. Antidiuretic hormone.
E. Prolactin.

The answer is E.

Dopamine inhibits the release of prolactin through the tuberoinfundibular pathway.

59. Based on biologic study, the level in the CSF of which of the following factors is inversely related to aggressive behavior?

A. Glutamate.
B. Histamine.
C. Neuropeptide Y.
D. 5-Hydroxyindoleacetic acid (5-HIAA), the major serotonin metabolite.

The answer is D.

The levels of 5-HIAA in the CSF correlate inversely with the frequency of aggression. Low levels of 5-HIAA are associated with aggressive behavior and suicide through violent methods.

Neurotransmitters and aggression:

Induction of aggression: Dopamine.

Inhibition of aggression: Norepinephrine, serotonin, GABA.

60. To which ion channel is GABA functionally related?

A. Sodium.
B. Potassium.
C. Chloride.
D. Calcium.

The answer is C.

GABA is functionally related to chloride channels that are regulated by GABA and other ligands. When GABA binds to its receptors, the chloride channels open, allowing more chloride influx into the cell and therefore increasing membrane polarization. Benzodiazepines bind to specific sites on GABA receptors and facilitate the effects of GABA (increased affinity of the GABA receptors for GABA).

61. All of the following disorders are associated with unstable triplet (trinucleotide) repeat sequences EXCEPT:

A. Huntington disease.
B. Fragile X syndrome.
C. Myotonic dystrophy.
D. Spinobulbar muscular atrophy.
E. Down syndrome.

The answer is E.

Down syndrome is trisomy 21, meaning that the patient has three replicates of chromosome 21, not a triplet repeat of nucleotides within a gene. All other conditions listed above are associated with unstable triplet repeat sequences.

62. What disorder in early life shows similar pathologic changes to those in Alzheimer disease?

A. Fragile X syndrome.
B. Prader-Willi syndrome.
C. Down syndrome.
D. Williams syndrome.

The answer is C.

The answer is Down syndrome. Both Alzheimer disease and Down syndrome are associated with defects in chromosome 21. Persons with Down syndrome who survive to early adulthood may present with histopathologic changes that are typical in Alzheimer disease (senile plaques and neurofibrillary tangles). There is also a clear familial association between the two diseases.

63. What is the pharmacologic treatment of choice for decreasing the craving for alcohol?

A. A benzodiazepine.
B. Naloxone.
C. Disulfiram.
D. Naltrexone.

The answer is D.

Objectives of pharmacologic treatment for alcoholism are to:

Reduce craving: Opioid antagonists (naltrexone, nalmefene), SSRIs (fluoxetine, citalopram), lithium, and bromocriptine.

Ease withdrawal: Benzodiazepines.

Create adverse conditioning: Disulfiram.

64. What is the mechanism of disulfiram to treat alcohol dependence?

A. Inhibiting central opiate receptors.
B. Augmenting GABA-mediated inhibition.
C. Increasing serum acetaldehyde levels.
D. Preventing the breakdown of ethanol in the blood.

The answer is C.

Disulfiram inhibits the alcohol-degrading enzyme acetaldehyde dehydrogenase and therefore raises blood levels of acetaldehyde, which can produce tachycardia, dyspnea, nausea, and vomiting. Disulfiram also inhibits dopamine β-hydroxylase.

Clinical effects of disulfiram last for up to 2 weeks after the last dose.

65. Data suggesting that alcoholism may be hereditary are based on studies of:

A. Siblings.
B. Parents.
C. Second-degree relatives.
D. Heterozygous twins.
E. Adopted siblings.

The answer is E.

Hereditary grounds for alcoholism were supported by studies of adopted siblings. The famous Danish adoption studies of familial determinants of alcoholism demonstrated that biologic sons of alcoholic persons were at higher risk of alcoholism than were biologic sons of nonalcoholic persons.

66. For what is the CAGE questionnaire used to screen?

A. Cocaine abuse.
B. Alcohol dependence.
C. Major depression.
D. General anxiety disorder.

The answer is B.

The CAGE questionnaire is used to screen patients for alcoholism; its letters stand for:

*C*ut: Have you ever felt you should cut down on your drinking?

*A*nnoyed: Have people annoyed you by criticizing your drinking?

*G*uilt: Have you ever felt guilty about your drinking?

*E*ye-opener: Have you ever taken a drink as your first act in the morning, to steady your nerves or get rid of a hangover?

67. A middle-aged chronic alcoholic male appears in the emergency room with disorientation and confusion. A neurologic examination shows ataxia and disconjugate eye movements. What is the diagnosis?

A. Bilateral subdural hematoma.
B. Wernicke encephalopathy.
C. Delirium tremens.
D. Pernicious anemia.

The answer is B.

Wernicke syndrome is a condition of acute onset and is completely reversible.

Korsakoff syndrome is chronic, and only 20% of patients may recover.

Symptoms of Wernicke syndrome (also called alcoholic encephalopathy) are:

- Ataxia.

- Confusion.
- Ophthalmoplegia (horizontal nystagmus, abducens paralysis, disconjugate eye movements, and gaze palsy).

Pathophysiology: Thiamine deficiency.

68. What is the maximum period for which cocaine can be detected in the urine?

A. Less than 6 hours.
B. Seven to 12 hours.
C. Two to 4 days.
D. One week.
E. Two weeks.

The answer is C.

Cocaine's metabolite, benzoylecgonine, can be detected in the urine 2 to 4 days after cocaine is used.

69. In the emergency room, a 25-year-old woman says that she is suicidal. She has been using crack cocaine in the past 5 days and feels depressed. She says that she had feelings of helplessness, hopelessness, and fatigue, with decreased appetite. What is the diagnosis?

A. Major depression.
B. Withdrawal syndrome.
C. Borderline personality disorder.
D. Anxiety disorder.

The answer is B.

Substance withdrawal syndrome can occur within hours to days after heavy use of a substance. It can be accompanied by significant mood changes. The acute onset of dysphoria, increased appetite, fatigue, psychomotor retardation or agitation, and sleep abnormalities (dreams, insomnia, or hypersomnia) that have followed cocaine use in the case described here are consistent with cocaine withdrawal, which again is usually paralleled by mood changes.

70. All of the following are clinical features of lysergic acid diethylamide (LSD) intoxication EXCEPT:

A. Paranoid ideation.
B. Depersonalization.
C. Tremor.
D. Synesthesia.
E. Pupillary constriction.

The answer is E.

Behavioral changes: Fear, anxiety, paranoid ideation, impaired judgment.

Perceptual changes: Perceptual changes in full wakefulness, depersonalization, derealization, illusions/hallucinations, and synesthesias.

Other: Pupil dilation.

Synesthesia: A sensation or hallucination caused by another sensation.

71. Which of the following is the most popular addictive substance in the United States?

A. Nicotine.
B. Alcohol.
C. Cocaine.
D. Heroin.
E. Phencyclidine (PCP).

The answer is A.

The most popular addictive substance is nicotine.

Among all the substance addictions, addiction to nicotine contributes most to premature death and disability, and is associated with the highest annual mortality.

72. A 24-year-old man who is well-known as a drug abuser to the emergency room staff is brought in by police after being found in a disoriented and confused state in the street. Upon examination, you find that the patient has mildly enlarged pupils, marked diaphoresis, lacrimation, and muscle ache. He yawns constantly during the examination and states that he has abdominal discomfort. What is your preliminary diagnosis?

A. Cocaine intoxication.
B. Cocaine withdrawal.
C. PCP intoxication.
D. Opiate intoxication.
E. Opiate withdrawal.

The answer is E.

Opioid withdrawal symptoms include disorientation, confusion, dysphoric mood, increased muscle tone, mildly enlarged pupils, increased blood pressure and heart rate, marked diaphoresis, piloerection, lacrimation (or rhinorrhea) and salivation, nausea or vomiting, diarrhea, yawning, fever, and insomnia.

73. A 28-year-old man is seen in the emergency room. He is comatose, with pinpoint pupils and decreased respiratory effort. His urine drug screen is positive for opiate. What is the immediate treatment of choice?

A. IV dextrose.
B. IV thiamine.
C. IV naloxone.
D. IV flumazenil.

The answer is C.

This is a case of severe opioid intoxication.

Symptoms of opioid intoxication: Pupillary constriction with drowsiness or coma, slurred speech, impairment in attention or memory, and pulmonary edema from central respiratory inhibition.

The pupils may be dilated from anoxia due to severe overdose.

Treatment of opioid intoxication: Naloxone 0.4 mg IV for respiratory depression or stupor.

Treatment of withdrawal: Clonidine or methadone.

The other choices shown are not for opioid intoxication. IV dextrose is for hypoglycemia, IV thiamine is for Wernicke syndrome, and IV flumazenil is for benzodiazepine intoxication.

74. Which of the following is not the clinical feature of PCP intoxication?

A. Nystagmus.
B. Hypotension or bradycardia.
C. Muscle rigidity.
D. Hyperacusis.
E. Numbness to pain.

The answer is B.

Signs of PCP intoxication:

1. Neurologic: Vertical or horizontal nystagmus, numbness, ataxia, dysarthria, muscle rigidity.
2. Autonomic: Hypertension, increased bronchial and salivary secretions.
3. Mental: Hyperacusis, labile affect, agitation, and assaultiveness.

PCP binds to N-methyl-D-aspartate subtype glutamate receptors.

75. According to the *Diagnostic and Statistical Manual of Mental Disorders, Fourth Edition* (DSM-IV), which of the following differentiates substance dependence from abuse?

A. Tolerance and withdrawal.
B. Social dysfunction.
C. A period of 12 months is required to make the diagnosis.
D. Interpersonal problems.

The answer is A.

The criteria for dependence include tolerance or withdrawal, which are not criteria for abuse.

76. What are the sleep abnormalities that may be detected with electroencephalography in depression?

A. Shortened latency of rapid eye movement (REM) sleep.
B. Decreased length of the first REM episode.
C. Decreased REM density.
D. Increased stage 4 sleep.

The answer is A.

In general, depressed patients have a reduced proportion of non-REM sleep and increased proportion of REM sleep.

1. Shortened REM latency.
2. Increased length of the first REM episode.
3. Increased REM density.
4. Decreased stage 4 sleep.
5. Increased awakening during the second half of the night.

77. All of the following are clinical features of posttraumatic stress disorder (PTSD) EXCEPT:

A. Re-experiencing of the event.
B. Increased arousal.
C. Avoidance of stimuli.
D. Duration of disturbance ranges from 1 week to 1 month.

The answer is D.

Key points in the diagnosis of PTSD:

Exposure to a traumatic event and:

Re-experiencing the event.

Increased arousal.

Avoidance of stimuli.

Numbing of general responsiveness.

Symptoms last longer than 1 month.

If the duration of the disturbance is less than 1 month, the disorder might be diagnosed as acute stress disorder.

78. All of the following diagnoses are categorized as somatoform disorders EXCEPT:

A. Briquet disease.
B. Pain disorder.
C. Body-dysmorphic disorder.
D. Munchausen syndrome.
E. Hypochondriasis.

The answer is D.

Munchausen syndrome is a factitious disorder with predominately physical signs and symptoms. It is not included in the category of somatoform disorders.

DSM-IV includes seven diagnoses under the category of somatoform disorders:

Somatization disorder (also known as Briquet syndrome), conversion disorder, hypochondriasis, pain disorder, body dysmorphic disorder, undifferentiated somatoform disorder, and somatoform disorder not otherwise specified.

79. The most common electrolyte imbalance seen in eating disorders is:

A. Hyponatremia.
B. Hypernatremia.
C. Hypokalemia.
D. Hyperkalemia.
E. Hypercalcemia.

The answer is C.

Hypokalemia.

When cardiac disturbance (anxiety, palpitation) is suspected in patients with an eating disorder, check the patient's serum potassium concentration.

80. A 30-year-old woman was referred by her internist for a consultation. She has repetitively presented herself with abdominal crises, paresthesias, and weakness. She has also had anxiety of sudden onset with severe mood swings, as well as frequent angry outbursts, and has sometimes complained of hearing voices. Her routine work up has been completely negative. Besides somatoform disorders, factitious disorders, and borderline personality disorders, what would you consider in your differential diagnosis?

A. Angina.
B. Acute intermittent porphyria.
C. Acute appendicitis.
D. Acute pancreatitis.

The answer is B.

Acute intermittent porphyria.

Symptoms: Colicky abdominal pain with nausea and vomiting, psychotic symptoms such as hallucinations, agitated depression, and polyneuropathy.

Acute intermittent porphyria has been estimated to be undiagnosed in 0.5% of psychiatric patients.

Test: Urine porphobilinogen and uroporphyrin.

81. A 30-year-old man presents with episodes of irresistible urges to sleep of sudden onset, and usually accompanied by a loss of muscle tone. It happened as often as four times a day and often lasts 10 to 20 minutes. The patient has also had vivid dreams while still conscious. What is the diagnosis?

A. Sleep terror.
B. Nightmare.
C. Narcolepsy.
D. Obstructive apnea.

The answer is C.

This is a typical case of narcolepsy. The DSM-IV criteria for this condition require that the episodes occur daily for more than 3 months, and present as one or both of the following:

1. Cataplexy (sudden loss of muscle tone, often precipitated by strong emotion), followed by entry into the REM stage of sleep within a few minutes of falling sleep;
2. Repeated intrusions of REM sleep into the transition between sleep and wakefulness (as manifested by hypnopompic or hypnagogic hallucinations or sleep paralysis).

Both nightmare disorder and sleep-terror disorder are parasomnias. Patients with nightmare disorder can remember the details of frightening dreams, whereas those with sleep-terror disorder cannot. In obstructive apnea, breathing is interrupted because of airway blockage (patients usually are obese), and respiratory effort continues.

82. Findings associated with diabetic neuropathy include all the following EXCEPT:

A. Numbness and pain.
B. Tremor.
C. Muscle weakness and atrophy.
D. Incontinence.
E. Postural hypotension.

The answer is B.

Diabetic neuropathy may present with sensory deficits (numbness and pain from mononeuropathy), autonomic neuropathy including incontinence, neurogenic bladder (with recurrent urinary tract infection), postural hypotension, and motor abnormalities that may result in muscle weakness and atrophy. Retinal and cranial nerve involvement (oculomotor, trochlear, and abducens nerves) by mononeuropathy simplex are very common. However, diabetic neuropathy does not cause tremor.

83. A 78-year-old white man presents with a complaint of gradual deterioration in memory and ability to take care of his bank accounts. His caregiver reports that he also mumbles to himself, laughs, or yells for no reason, and easily becomes agitated. The patient's gait is impaired. He has been wheelchair-bound for the past 2 years. A computed tomographic scan of the head shows generalized atrophy. The patient's CSF shows 51 white blood cells (WBCs)/mm^3, of which 46 are lymphocytes. The CSF protein is 112 mg/dL. The γ-globulin concentration in the patient's CSF is elevated. Oligoclonal bands are present upon protein electrophoresis of the CSF. The most important next test is:

A. Immunoblot detection of prion protein (scrapie) PrPSc.
B. EEG.
C. MRI.
D. Fluorescent treponemal antibody absorption test (FTA-ABS).
E. CSF morphology.

The answer is D.

This is a typical case of late neurosyphilis, which presents with dementia and other psychiatric symptoms. The patient may also have both tabes dorsalis and taboparesis as the cause of his wheelchair-bound status. His CSF has an elevated WBC count (predominantly lymphocytes) and protein concentration, increased γ-globulin concentration, and presence of oligoclonal protein bands. The next test done should be a treponemal confirmatory test such as blood FTA-ABS or microhemagglutination-*Treponema pallidum* (MHA-TP).

Immunoblot detection of PrPSc is a test for Creutzfeldt-Jakob disease.

EEG and MRI are nonspecific for neurosyphilis.

CSF morphology may be helpful for the diagnosis of lymphoma of the CNS, but not for neurosyphilis.

84. All of the following pathologic findings are characteristic of idiopathic Parkinson disease EXCEPT:

A. Loss of pigmentation in the substantia nigra.
B. Neurofibrillary degeneration in the substantia nigra.
C. Cell loss in the substantia nigra.
D. Cell loss in the globus pallidus and putamen.
E. Presence of eosinophilic intraneural inclusion granules.

The answer is B.

The pathologic features of idiopathic parkinsonism include loss of pigmentation and cells in the substantia nigra and other brainstem centers, cell loss in the globus pallidus and putamen, and the presence of eosinophilic intraneural inclusion granules (Lewy bodies) in the basal ganglia, brainstem, spinal cord, and sympathetic ganglia.

Neurofibrillary tangles as well as neuritic plaques and granulovacuolar degeneration are typical histopathologic features seen in Alzheimer dementia.

85. A 25-year-old woman complains of progressive numbness and weakness in the shoulders and arms. Physical examination shows deficient sensation of pain and temperature in the shoulders and both upper extremities. Touch and vibration sensations, however, are preserved. Deep tendon reflexes are absent. Muscle atrophy is noticed in the patient's forearms and hands. The most likely diagnosis can be confirmed by:

A. MRI.
B. Serum vitamin B_{12} assay.
C. CSF examination.
D. Muscle biopsy.
E. Serum creatine phosphokinase (CPK) assay.

The answer is A.

This is a case of anterior spinal cord lesion. Possible etiologies include syringomyelia, spinal compression, and occlusion of the anterior spinal artery. Pain and temperature appreciation are impaired below the level of the lesion, by involvement of the lateral spinothalamic tract. In addition, weakness or paralysis of muscles supplied by the involved segments of the cord results from damage to motor neurons in the anterior horn. However, there is relative preservation of posterior column function such as the sensations of touch and vibration. The best procedure for viewing the spinal cord pathology in such a case is MRI.

The symptoms do not indicate vitamin B_{12} deficiency.

CSF examination may show nonspecific change, but is not helpful for locating a morphologic change in the cord.

Muscle biopsy and measurement of the serum CPK level are useful in diagnosing neuromyopathy.

86. A 41-year-old man complains of pain about the ear, difficulty in closing his right eye, and drooping of his right face. He finds that his right ear is very sensitive to loud, low-frequency sounds. When a small spoonful of sugar is applied to the right side of his tongue, he says that it tastes like sand. Physical examination shows right-sided weakness of both the upper and lower face. The patient's symptoms started 3 days ago. The most likely diagnosis is:

A. Stroke.
B. Diabetic neuropathy.
C. Chronic migraine.
D. Idiopathic Bell palsy.
E. Tic douloureux.

The answer is D.

Bell palsy is a facial weakness of the lower motor neuron type. It is caused by idiopathic facial nerve involvement outside the CNS. Ear pain is common. Impairment of taste, lacrimation, or hyperacusis can also be present. The onset can be abrupt. The symptoms can progress in hours to a day.

The lower motor neuron symptom rules out stroke, which involves upper motor neurons in the CNS.

Diabetic neuropathy rarely involves the trigeminal nerve. There are no other symptoms in this case that indicate diabetic neuropathy.

Although chronic migraine can present with acute exacerbation, the clinical context of this case is not consistent with such a diagnosis.

Tic douloureux (trigeminal neuralgia) presents with typical pain in areas of the face supplied by the second and third divisions of the trigeminal nerve. No facial weakness is found on examination.

87. In radiologic examination of the brain, CT is preferred over MRI when:

A. A good differentiation of white from gray matter is essential.
B. The presumed lesion is in the posterior fossa or brainstem.
C. Acute hemorrhage is suspected.
D. The patient is pregnant.
E. The patient suffers from claustrophobia.

The answer is C.

Advantages of CT:

1. Detection of acute bleeding (less than 24 to 72 hours old).
2. Suitable for patients with metallic implants.
3. No need for a prolonged stay in a narrow space (which may induce claustrophobia).

Advantages of MRI:

1. Excellent soft tissue contrast reveals white matter.
2. Excellent imaging of the posterior fossa and brainstem.
3. Preferable in pregnancy.

88. A positive Romberg test indicates dysfunction of the:

A. Dorsal columns.
B. Cerebellar vermis.
C. Muscles of the lower extremities.
D. Vestibular system.
E. Vascular supply of the lower extremities.

The answer is A.

Neurologic tests:

Romberg test: Dorsal column function.

Stance and gait: Cerebellar vermis function.

Muscle strength: Muscles of the lower extremities.

Nylen-Barany (Dix-Hallpike) maneuver: Vestibular system function.

Doppler ultrasonography: Vascular supply of the lower extremities.

89. Characteristic clinical features and examination findings in cases of hypertensive encephalopathy include all of the following EXCEPT:

A. Headache and vomiting.
B. Seizures.
C. Papilledema, retinal arteriolar spasm, retinal hemorrhages, and exudates.
D. CT scan usually shows a normal brain.
E. MRI T2-weighted phase study shows low-density areas suggestive of edema.

The answer is D.

In hypertensive encephalopathy, both CT and T2-weighted MRI scans show low-density areas suggestive of edema in the posterior regions of hemispheric white matter.

90. Which of the following results of hearing assessment indicates conductive hearing loss?

A. Rinne test: Air conduction as fast as bone conduction.
B. Weber test: Sound perceived as coming from normal ear.
C. Weber test: Sound perceived as coming from midline.
D. Weber test: Sound perceived as coming from affected ear.
E. Rinne test: Bone conduction slower than air conduction on affected side.

The answer is D.

Normal:

Weber test: Sound perceived as coming from midline.

Rinne test: Air conduction faster than bone conduction.

Sensorineural hearing loss:

Weber test: Sound perceived as coming from normal ear.

Rinne test: Air conduction faster than bone conduction.

Conductive hearing loss:

Weber test: Sound perceived as coming from affected ear.

Rinne test: Bone conduction faster than air conduction on affected side.

91. Clinical findings in myasthenia gravis include all of the following EXCEPT:

A. Slowly progressive course.
B. Diplopia, ptosis, dysarthria, and dysphagia.
C. The weakness does not conform to the distribution of any single nerve.
D. Pupillary responses are often affected.
E. Persistent activity of a muscle group leads to temporarily increased weakness, with restoration of strength after a brief rest.

The answer is D.

Myasthenia gravis affects neuromuscular transmission in skeletal muscle. The postsynaptic receptor involved in this process is a nicotinic-type acetylcholine receptor. Pupillary responses are instead controlled by the autonomic system. The postsynaptic receptor in the parasympathetic system is the muscarinic receptor, which differs from the nicotinic receptor, and the postsynaptic receptors in the sympathetic system are adrenoceptors. Thus, myasthenia gravis does not affect pupillary responses.

92. A boy understands that a tall cup and a bowl may contain the same volume of water. When asked why he likes to visit his uncle, he answered: "My uncle is lonely." When asked why dad has to work every day, he answered: "So he makes money and so we have the house and food." According to Jean Piaget's theory of development, this boy is likely to be in what age range?

A. 0 to 2 years.
B. 2 to 7 years.
C. 7 to 11 years.
D. 11 to 15 years.
E. 15 to 18 years.

The answer is C.

The preoperational stage occurs from the ages of 7 to 11 and is characterized by the appropriate use of logic. Children start to understand the concept of conservation (water in a tall cup has the same volume as water in a bowl). Children also start to eliminate egocentrism and develop the ability to understand someone else's point of view.

93. A child constantly is concerned about the actual physical location of her mother. She frequently runs back to check on mother while she is playing. She becomes whining and moody when her mother is devoted to her own work. According to Mahler's separation-individuation theory, what is likely the girl's age?

A. 0 to 2 months.
B. 2 to 5 months.
C. 5 to 10 months.
D. 10 to 18 months.
E. 18 to 24 months.

The answer is E.

Rapprochement is the best known of Margaret Mahler's six developmental stages: Normal autism (birth to 2 months); symbiosis (2 to 5 months); differentiation (5 to 10 months); practicing (10 to 18 months); rapprochement (18 to 24 months); and object constancy (2 to 5 years).

94. Which of the following agents may decrease lithium levels?

A. Angiotensin-converting enzyme inhibitors.
B. Theophylline.
C. Fluoxetine.
D. Ibuprofen.
E. Spironolactone.

The answer is B.

The rest of the answers are agents that may increase lithium levels.

95. In the stage of development between age 18 to 24 months, children constantly are concerned about the actual physical location of their mothers, and have great need for maternal love. This stage is termed as what and endorsed by whom?

A. "Preoperational" by Jean Piaget.
B. "Transitional" by Donald W. Winnicott.
C. "Rapprochement" by Margaret Mahler.
D. "Self-object" by Heinz Kohut.
E. "Toddler" by Hans Asperger.

The answer is C.

This is a typical description of rapprochement in Margaret Mahler's separation-individuation theory.

96. The following receptors are all constructed with a single long peptide and have seven transmembrane domains EXCEPT:

A. D2.
B. 5-HT3.
C. D3.
D. Opioid receptor μ.
E. NE α1.

The answer is B.

The single unit receptor with seven transmembrane domains implies a G-protein coupled receptor. All 5-HT receptors, except 5-HT3, are G-protein coupled receptors. The serotonin 5-HT3 receptor is an excitatory, directly coupled, multiple unit, Na^+-K^+ channel receptor. Dopamine receptors, opioid receptors, and norepinephrine receptors are all G-protein coupled receptors.

97. The following are schneiderian first rank symptoms EXCEPT:

A. Voices heard commenting on one's actions.
B. Thought broadcast.
C. Imposed impulses.
D. Delusional perception.
E. Tactile hallucination.

The answer is E.

There are three first rank symptoms that are associated with hallucination: Audible thoughts, voices heard arguing, and voices heard commenting on one's actions. All three are auditory hallucinations. There is no other form of hallucination that is a schneiderian first rank symptom.

98. The following are associated with a good prognosis in schizophrenia EXCEPT:

A. Late onset age.
B. Insidious onset.
C. Confusion at the height of the psychotic episode.
D. Female gender.
E. Positive symptoms.

The answer is B.

Acute onset, not insidious onset, is a factor associated with good prognosis.

99. The following neurophysiologic changes are believed to occur during the process of ECT EXCEPT:

A. Downregulation of norepinephrine and serotonin receptors.
B. Increase of the extracellular serotonin and norepinephrine concentration.
C. Rise in seizure threshold.
D. Increase of brain derived neurotrophic factor.
E. Increase in neurogenesis in the hippocampus.

The answer is A.

ECT causes upregulation of norepinephrine and serotonin receptors, which is the same effect seen with long-term use of antidepressants.

100. Which of the following neurotransmitter receptors is considered an "excitatory" receptor?

A. GABA A.
B. Dopamine D2.
C. Dopamine D1.
D. Opioid μ.
E. Norepinephrine *α*2.

The answer is C.

Receptors for neurotransmitters are categorized into either excitatory or inhibitory. When activated by proper neurotransmitters, excitatory receptors promote depolarization and increase the likelihood of action potential, while inhibitory receptors can produce hyperpolarization and decrease the likelihood of action potential. All GABA receptors are inhibitory receptors. Among dopamine receptors, D1 and D5 are excitatory, while D2, D3, and D4 are inhibitory receptors. Opioid receptors are all inhibitory. Norepinephrine α1 and β are excitatory, and α2 is inhibitory.

APPENDIX II

In Preparation for the Board: Practical Tips

This book is designed to help the organization of a thorough study as well as to provide a last-minute grasp of information for the Board. For the tedious task of preparing for the Board, we believe an intensive study for a period of at least 4 months is needed. However, commitment to giving time alone is not enough. A correct and efficient strategy is essential to master a vast volume of knowledge. From surveys and our personal experience, we found the best strategies are usually unconventional. Reading a standard textbook was found to be the least efficient in test preparation. The popular strategy of doing an assimilated test is usually insufficient. If you are determined to do it once and do it right, our advice is:

DO read repetitively.

DO study real cases.

DO study daily or nearly daily.

DO ask and teach.

DO read *Psychiatry for the Boards,* 2nd edition.

DO NOT follow a textbook in sequence of chapters.

DO NOT depend on rigorous study for a short period of time.

DO NOT rely only on assimilated tests.

DO NOT be overly obsessed with cutting-edge research data.

DO NOT omit psychosocial theories.

The following is a suggested plan for a 4-month/4-round approach.

First Round

10 weeks (16 to 7 weeks before the examination).

Task: To assess vulnerable areas, study unfamiliar subjects, and prepare for building blocks of knowledge.

Suggested approach:

- Read *Psychiatry for the Boards,* 2nd edition. This initial reading gives you the scope of knowledge required for the examination and helps indicate the kind of material you will need. We do not suggest answering the Board-type questions during the first round.
- Collect and organize the necessary study material.
- Make a study plan for the following 10 weeks. You may want to digest several (three to five) intensive chapters in those areas in which your training program may have been relatively weak. Remember that although many residency programs claim certain strengths in their training, the ABPN requires a balanced clinical knowledge and skill set.
- Study every day. Daily study is proven to be superior to periodic rigorous cramming. You will also find more weak areas while studying. Make notes and look for the material required for further study.
- Do not follow the sequential plan of any textbook. Following a textbook by chapter sequentially is very boring and most tiring. We also suggest case study. Select patients from your practice, and study the relevant chapters. This is a very powerful approach. With the vivid case in front of you, you will never forget the material you absorbed while treating this patient.
- Highlight your material. Make notes. Use mnemonics.
- If you have any peers who are preparing for the same examination, we suggest no communication at this stage. Communicating too early may provoke anxiety and distract you from concentrated study.

Second Round

4 weeks (6 to 3 weeks before the examination).

Task: To reorganize the material, trim the already mastered subjects, and acknowledge necessary trivial facts and numbers.

Suggested approach:

- If you have not read this book in your first round, this is an appropriate time to finish.
- Answer the questions in this book.
- Reorganize your material. If there is any major area of material that you did not have time to digest in the first round, you will probably not be able to complete it. Do not attempt to do so; you will never be competent in every area of psychiatry. To pass the examination, you need only one thing: The total score.
- Plan your study for the next 4 weeks. It is essential to budget most of your time for reviewing those areas you already studied and identified for further study in your first round. Remember, in order to increase your score, you have to master the knowledge in a particular area, not merely acquaint yourself with it. Too often test-takers are frustrated when given a question that looks familiar but to which they cannot ascertain the right answer.
- Work on the second-round tasks. Do not extend your first round into this time period.
- Put aside a small amount of material that you need to read one more time before the examination.
- Consider communicating with your peers. This is the stage at which you should know where your stand and what you needed to study further.

Third Round

2 weeks (2 to 1 week before the examination).

Task: To sharpen the learned knowledge, memorize necessary trivial facts and numbers, and familiarize yourself with the test format.

Suggested approach:

- If you haven't read this book, this is the last chance, and you should read it as a new book. Otherwise, we suggest skipping the already well-learned items, and focusing on those you are still unfamiliar with.
- Review highlighted and checked material, including those brought to your attention from discussion with peers.

- Do not spend more time in learning any new topics, unless they are very short and you feel they are very important.
- Write down a few mnemonics for last-minute study.

Fourth Round

2 days (2 to 1 day before the examination).

Task: Last-minute cram.

Suggested approach:

- Consider taking time off work.
- Read *Psychiatry for the Boards*, 2nd edition, one more time. However, if you have not read this book yet, we suggest focusing on material you are already working on. You probably already learned enough and it is too late to start any new book.
- Review mnemonics.
- You should not leave intensive study to this stage.
- Do not study the night before the examination. A serious 6-hour examination is not only about knowledge. The challenge is to give a knowledge-powered performance. Consider engaging in light aerobic exercise and listening to soothing music. Rest well and replenish your energy.

Enjoy your study and perform well on your real test.

William W. Wang, M.D., Ph.D.
Wen-Hui Cai, M.D., Ph.D.

INDEX

Index

Index